This dynamic,
proven program
shows you how to:

- Slow the aging process with the kind of exercise that "buys years"

- Dispense with 15 myths about physical fitness that simply are not true

- Vary your meals for maximum nutrition

- Use your pulse as a built-in "speedometer" that tells you how much exercise your body needs for optimum fitness

- Fool the eating habit and halt "creeping obesity" with a simple 100-calorie adjustment

- Improve a bad back or sagging stomach and get other problem areas back in shape

- Use your morning shower to exercise your hands, wrists, arms, shoulders, and chest

- Improve your bustline or muscle tone without exotic developers or exercises

- Find out which tailor-made plan will give you the best results in the shortest time

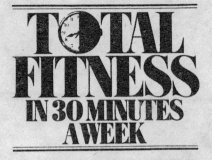

TOTAL FITNESS
IN 30 MINUTES A WEEK

**LAURENCE E. MOREHOUSE, Ph.D.
and LEONARD GROSS**

POCKET BOOKS

New York   London   Toronto   Sydney   Tokyo

Drawings by Judy Francis

POCKET BOOKS, a division of Simon & Schuster Inc.
1230 Avenue of the Americas, New York, NY 10020

Published by arrangement with Simon and Schuster
Library of Congress Catalog Card Number: 74-16116

ISBN: 0-671-68349-7

First Pocket Books printing February 1976

20   19   18   17

POCKET and colophon are trademarks of
Simon & Schuster Inc.

Printed in the U.S.A.

Our thanks to those men and women who voluntarily exercised to exhaustion in physiology laboratories to establish that a desirable level of fitness can be achieved without strain and sweat.

FOR THELMA AND JACKIE

PREFACE

by Leonard Gross

The temperature was above ninety. Our set score stood at 5–4. Suddenly, my opponent excused himself, walked from the tennis court and began to drink copiously at the water fountain.

I walked over. "Has the sun gotten to you?" I said. "You, of all people, drinking during exercise."

"Forget it," he replied. "We know now that it's not just the salt you lose but the water you lose that makes you tired. Today you replace water while exercising."

My opponent was my physician. Twenty-five years ago, as a half-miler and captain of the UCLA track team, he never drank while exercising.

The episode made me wonder whether there might be other rules we had all religiously followed that were no longer valid. I thought it might make an interesting magazine article, if true. A few phone calls led me to Dr. Laurence E. Morehouse, professor of exercise physiology at UCLA, founding director of the university's Human Performance Laboratory. When I explained my quest, he laughed.

"You've hit a gold mine," he said. "Come on over." I found an unpretentious office and an unprepossessing man whom I took for fifty-two. I later learned he was sixty. In less than an hour, he demolished every notion I had harbored about fitness, conditioning and personal maintenance—including diet and weight loss. And he sizably enlarged my objective.

"Have you ever written a book?" I ventured.

"I've written twelve," he replied.

All twelve, it developed, were textbooks. Dr. Morehouse had never written a book for the general public. He agreed to write one with me.

A year has passed. The book is finished. And I am confirmed in my suspicion that there is a time lag of twenty-five years between the development of knowledge and its dissemination to the public.

In the world of physiology, Professor Morehouse is an oracle. His book on the subject is the standard text in colleges and universities throughout the world. He is the author of the sections on exercise and physical conditioning in the *Encyclopaedia Britannica,* the *Encyclopedia Americana,* the *Encyclopedia of Sports Medicine* and the *Encyclopedia of Physical Education.* When America's astronauts orbit the earth in Skylab, they exercise on a machine invented by Dr. Morehouse, according to a system he devised. It is an ingenious system, adaptable to earthlings, yet, until now, it has not been widely available to the public.

The system is revolutionary, in that it breaks with the existing order. But there is nothing violent about it. To the contrary, what severs the Morehouse system from all others is its gentle approach to fitness—and weight control as well. There's no need to punish yourself, he argues. The proof is in this book.

I had never imagined I would be involved in such a book. My field is man's social, not his physical, condition. But I have a penchant for keeping fit. We have epic arguments in our house about how to do that. One of our great arguments concerns diet. My bride of twenty-three years, who was a college queen, engages periodically in heroic bouts of abstinence. Dr. Morehouse considers the loss of more than a pound a week suicidal. He advocates a "wide-variety diet." He maintains that we need every kind of food. Quick-loss diets are rip-offs, he demonstrates, injurious and ineffective. His formula for permanent weight loss is a tolerable increase in physical activity and a tiny reduction in calories.

Dr. Morehouse's theories are amply documented by research spanning forty years. Much of his work is carried on in conjunction with physicians at UCLA, the National Aeronautics and Space Administration, and other medical-research units. But because I'm a reporter by training, I needed a further increment of evidence before I could commit myself to the book. I had to try the theories myself.

I not only learned that just about everything I had been doing was wrong, I found out that I was doing far more than I needed to. I had been spending forty-five minutes a day, four days a week, divided between nineteen different exercises. The workouts were so arduous that I approached them with dread. I often took shortcuts. Sometimes I failed to work out, either because I didn't have the time or because I didn't have the inclination. Often the lack of inclination made it seem that I didn't have the time. My guilt was sizable, and the results were spotty. Dr. Morehouse proposed that I cut my exercises to four, my days to three, and my "sets" to one, instead of the two I'd been doing. Each of these sessions now takes ten minutes, instead of forty-five—a total of thirty minutes a week instead of three hours. It's been some time now since I missed a workout. I seem to be significantly more energetic. I can work longer. I'm more alert in the evening. I'm not undone by a short sleep. I last better on the tennis court. I'm beating opponents who had always beaten me. Inasmuch as my tennis skills haven't changed in the last year, I have to ascribe this turn to an increased endurance and ability to retrieve. I'm simply getting to balls that used to go for winners—a fact my opponents have remarked.

At the outset of our collaboration, Dr. Morehouse and I agreed that we were writing a book for the man or woman who wanted to live a long, healthy life and, as the professor put it, "not be so damned tired at the end of the day." Larry Morehouse's message is that you don't have to kill yourself to stay in shape. You can look younger, feel better and probably live longer by exercising, his way, for thirty minutes a week.

CONTENTS

	Preface	9
I	Fitness Is a Piece of Cake	17
II	Fifteen Fitness Myths	34
III	Fit for What?	55
IV	What Happens When You Do— and If You Don't	82
V	How To Lose Weight Forever Without Torturing Yourself in the Process	98
VI	The Theory of Heart-rated Exercise	132
VII	All About Your Pulse	147
VIII	Your Pulse Test	160
IX	Minimum Maintenance	173
X	How to Acquire a Reserve of Fitness in Thirty Minutes a Week	190
XI	Three Short Steps to Fitness	211
XII	Finishing Touches	238

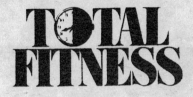

TOTAL FITNESS

1

Fitness Is a Piece of Cake

I hate to exercise. I always have. In high school, I was the gym-class rebel. When the rest of the class did calisthenics with their arms, I mimicked them with my fingers. My friends thought I was hilarious. My gym teacher didn't think so. One day he called me into his office and said, "I notice that you like to lead your little group. I'm going to give you the opportunity to lead the entire class."

It was one thing to be a cut-up. It was another to be a fool. I spent the weekend reading books on physical conditioning. When the teacher called on me the following Monday, I was ready. From then on, I led the class in calisthenics, and he sat in his office and read the newspaper.

I didn't know it at the time, but that assignment shaped my life. For the last forty-three years, I have studied human performance and how it can be enhanced. I've worked with world-class champions to improve their speed or power or skills. I've helped corporate executives develop their energy and concentration. I've designed a program to maintain the fitness of America's astronauts in space, on the moon and during their eventual trip to Mars. But nothing I have done in this interval has in any way changed my bias against structured exercise; to the contrary, what I've learned has only deepened it.

Most Americans share my bias—women in particular. Newspapers and magazines make much of statistics indicating that millions of Americans are on a fitness kick. That isn't really true. The figures, from a survey made for the President's Council on Physical Fitness and Sport, show that fifty-five percent of the nation's adults engage in some form of exercise. But when the activities themselves are analyzed, it's apparent that at least eighty percent of the adult population isn't exercising sufficiently or properly to arrest physiological decay.

In their resistance to exercise, Americans show a certain amount of commendable intuitive sense. Exercise, as it is generally taught and practiced, is not simply boring; it is punitive, dangerous and ineffective.

HOW EXERCISE BECAME SUCH A BORE

Calisthenics originated in Sweden during the nineteenth century. Swedish landowners found the sight of their stooped and sagging peasants offensive; they investigated physical drills to improve the peasants' posture and counteract the effects of work. They wanted the peasants to bear themselves like soldiers. As a consequence, calisthenic drills and movements became militaristic: by the numbers, shoulders back. That's not just philosophically offensive, it's physiologically harmful. Precise, geometric movements are unnatural and inefficient; movement should be accomplished in a flowing manner and in a circular plane. As to posture, holding the chest up, shoulders back and head erect puts an extra burden on the muscles. The straight, flat back esteemed by the military is a painful back. The best position for the shoulders is hanging loose to the sides, not braced to a point that puts a harmful weight on the spine. The vertical posture is not meant to be exaggerated; man was constructed to be only somewhat upright.

Exercise programs are often so rigorous that those who attempt them are injured. The goals of fitness are placed beyond the average person's reach. The mystique fostered by the fitness cult encourages the belief that good physical condition comes slowly, that work to exhaustion is necessary, that the process requires special equipment, space, supervision and an abundance of time. Men should look like Tarzan. Women should resemble his Jane. It's all nonsense.

The science of physical fitness concerns itself primarily with athletes. Physical-fitness "experts" are usually athletic coaches. Books on jogging are written by track coaches. The training they impose on the public reflects their orientation. But an athlete is a different person, psychologically and physiologically, from the nonathlete. Athletes will take the time to train. They will sacrifice social pleasures, endure discomfort, even punish themselves in order to create the tolerances required for record-breaking performances. These attributes do not characterize the majority of people.

A secondary emphasis of the science of fitness is

in therapy for persons recuperating from illness. In therapy, you concentrate on the injured or diseased part, rather than on the body as a whole. Those fitness programs that focus on isolated body parts stem from a therapeutic orientation. Once again, the objectives and techniques of exercise have almost no bearing on the needs of normal people.

So we find exercise concentrated at two extremes of the human condition—superbly fit athletes at one end, and hospital patients on the mend at the other. In the center of the spectrum are the overwhelming majority of nonathletic Americans who are healthy and capable of exertion and yet do almost no exercise at all.

Our cultural values reinforce their lassitude. We esteem those who can ride rather than walk and who can sit rather than stand. The higher one rises in the hierarchy, the greater one's comfort and ease. Wealthy golfers drive golf carts. We hire athletes to perform for us so that we can enjoy sports vicariously. We buy expensive, fuel-costly devices promoted as energy "savers." They're not saving us a thing; they're depriving us of the movement and exertion we need to live an energetic life.

HOW TO SLOW THE AGING PROCESS

If I have learned one thing in my years of study, it is that the fountain of youth for which Ponce de Leon searched in vain was right inside his body. Exercise is the means to an alert, vigorous and lengthy life. Inactivity will kill you.

A few years ago, an engineer at the National Aeronautics and Space Administration answered an invitation my group had tendered key members of the space program to take a physiological test. We found that he had an undernourished heart muscle, and advised him to start a reconditioning program. But he was too busy to exercise. Two weeks later, a neighbor's house caught fire. The engineer rushed over to help carry belongings to the street. In the confusion of the fire, no one saw his distress. Later, he was found dead in the gutter. The engineer had the kind of heart condition that responds well to exercise. We were convinced that mere minutes of exercise during that two-week interval could have saved his life—if only by establishing a level of tolerance he would have known not to exceed.

The more common signs of physiological aging are less dramatic but no less remorseless—infirmity, feebleness, frailness, sallowness, low energy and loss of the fight against gravity. Physiological aging literally pulls you down; your height diminishes, your body stoops, you dodder.

But while chronological age is invariable, *physiological* age has a variable of thirty years. Suppose you are fifty. You can have the outward appearance and internal system of a sixty-five-year-old—or a thirty-five-year-old. It's entirely up to you. An inactive life is a slow form of suicide. The right kind of exercise buys years.

There was a toxicologist in his fifties at NASA who, when I first met him, looked like an obese old man. Six months later he began a weight-loss program. He lost thirty pounds, but he was flabby and his flesh hung from him. He felt weak. Then we put him on an exercise program. Within five months, he became so well conditioned that he joined me in a scuba diving course. He easily kept up with the younger men in the class, and became a qualified diver.

QUIET AND SHOCK: THE LETHAL EXTREMES

The biological basis for human health behavior lies in the principle that slight change is necessary for all life. If you put a single-cell creature such as an amoeba or a paramecium in a vessel that contains the ideal environment—just the right amount of light and warmth, the proper acidity or alkalinity, all the food it needs—and keep the environment free of all abrasives such as noise, vibrations and pollutants, the creature will soon die. If you put another single-cell creature into an environment with multiple, persistent changes of a great magnitude, that creature won't survive either. But if you put a third creature into an environment with occasional, slight changes, it will survive a normal length of time.

How often we've heard compulsive people say, "I'm going to work hard and play hard." The organism may never recover from such overindulgence. By contrast, we all know someone who, approaching retirement, boasts, "I'm going to get myself a rocking chair and a bunch of novels and enjoy life by doing nothing." These are the symptoms that antecede early death in retirement of apparently healthy people.

The extreme of quietude is just as lethal as the extreme of biological shock. Both insult the system.

If we could play eighteen holes of golf or two sets of tennis every day, we'd have to do little more to stay in shape. Few of us can do that. We haven't got the time or the opportunity or the money or even the inclination. *Ergo,* exercise.

But exercise shouldn't be hateful, punishing, interminable and dull. It needn't be any of these.

Fitness is a piece of cake. You can achieve and maintain fitness in just twice the amount of time you require to brush your teeth. You need about fifteen minutes a week to brush your teeth. You need about thirty minutes a week to be fit.

EVERYTHING YOU DON'T NEED TO DO

Before I tell you what you can do with those thirty minutes, let me tell you what you won't have to do to stay fit.

You don't have to kill yourself. You will never exercise to the point of exhaustion.

You don't have to feel guilty if you fall off the wagon on any given day. If you just haven't got it, don't worry about it. Quit exercising, and try again tomorrow or the next day.

You don't have to eliminate foods or beverages of any kind. Diets that restrict the kinds of foods you can eat or that grossly curtail your intake are inhuman, injurious and doomed to fail. If weight loss is your goal, you can do it on a *wide-variety diet* that we'll talk about extensively farther on. You'll also learn why you may actually be required to *gain* weight at times in order to assure yourself of an eventual permanent weight loss.

You don't have to run a certain distance, or race against a clock or lift so much weight so many times.

You don't have to feel that your goal is unachievable. It will be a goal that reflects *your* condition, *your* capacity for physical effort and *your* needs and objectives.

And you don't have to spend a penny. There are no gimmicks to buy or pills to swallow. There's no special equipment to use or wear. You can perform your program in your underwear. All you'll need is a watch or a clock with a sweep second hand.

A DIFFERENT APPROACH TO FITNESS

Obviously, a program like this would have to be different from any previous fitness program. It is.

All previous programs measure the work you produce—the distance you run or the speed at which you run it or the number of times you can accomplish a specific task. *This* program ignores exterior accomplishments in favor of interior results. *This* system is interested in only one thing—the effect you produce on your body. *You* regulate that effect entirely. *You* produce exactly the response to effort that you wish and require.

The problem with previous exercise systems is that they assign tasks that either are too difficult at the outset or become easier and easier to perform. It's all very well to run or swim faster or farther, but if your internal system is not responding to the right degree you're not achieving fitness.

Previous systems program you into specific tasks. This system offers you your choice of any activity you find enjoyable. All that matters is that the activity churn your system to a level appropriate for *your* particular circumstances.

You monitor that activity. You set the pace in terms of what the activity is doing to your circulo-respiratory system—your heart and vessels and lungs. You do this by taking your pulse—which you'll shortly learn to do.

Your program is based on principles employed in the Apollo program to prepare America's astronauts for life in outer space, and to monitor their activity once there. I helped to create that program while a member of NASA's metabolic-management committee.

It was our job to monitor the amount of energy each astronaut was using so that he didn't exceed either his own capacity or that of his life-support system. We were also concerned that no astronaut work beneath his capacity while he was in space. The Apollo program was an expensive project; we wanted our money's worth.

HEART RATE: A LOUD AND CLEAR
SIGNAL OF EFFORT

When a man works on the surface of the moon, three signals indicate the extent of his effort: his consumption of oxygen, his body heat and his heart rate. The measurement of oxygen consumption is about as revealing as watching the fuel gauge on your automobile. The gauge tells you how much gas you have left, but it doesn't say anything about the efficiency or condition of the engine. The temperature of the fluids in your system that cools the astronaut inside his space suit tells you how much heat he's giving off, which gives you an idea of the amount of energy he's using. But it takes ten to fifteen minutes to obtain these figures and decide what has happened ten or fifteen minutes earlier. By then it may be too late to make an adjustment. The same problem exists in measuring oxygen consumption.

The third signal is the heart rate. It's loud and clear.

It takes a while for the body to heat up. Oxygen usage occurs over a prolonged period. But heart rate is an immediately available indicator of the level of physical effort as of that very moment.

If an astronaut is working too fast, a doctor in Houston monitoring the mission can tell him to slow down. If the astronaut's heart rate is below what has been gauged acceptable for that task and that astronaut, the doctor can advise the astronaut that he could work a little harder without impairing his condition.

It was the problem of maintaining the fitness of astronauts during prolonged space flights that turned my thinking around. We know that a man who does nothing for a month will lose eighty percent of his physical condition. An astronaut who did little or nothing active in Skylab or on trips to distant planets would quickly become too weak to perform his mission. How to keep him fit? It occurred to me that traditional fitness programs wouldn't work. Each time he did an exercise, the astronaut would do it more easily. His body wouldn't be exercised sufficiently. Making the exercise progressively more arduous was helpful, but it still wouldn't tell us whether the workout was sufficient—or too strenuous. It became evident to me that exercise should not be controlled on the basis of time, distance, physical load or other external scales, but on the degree of physiological effort as indicated by physiological signals.

NASA adopted a program based on these principles in 1965. Its efficacy was confirmed eight years later, when three U.S. astronauts returned from a twenty-eight-day mission in Skylab. It was thought that they might have to be carried from their capsule in stretchers. But they had maintained an activity schedule I helped develop for them, based on physiological effort. They walked away from the capsule, a little wobbly, but under their own power.

The physiological signal used by the astronauts

to monitor their maintenance programs was their heart rate. Using heart rate to monitor exercise in ordinary people is a research bonus of the space program.

WHAT YOUR PULSE SIGNALS

Heart rate and pulse rate, technically, are separate phenomena. But the difference, for our purpose, is not significant. Your pulse tells you how fast your heart is beating.

We all know that pulse rate is important. When you go to a doctor's office for a checkup, there are three things his nurse almost invariably does: she takes your temperature, weighs you and takes your pulse. If you've ever spent any time in a hospital, one of the first things you become aware of is that people are taking your pulse all day long. They awaken you in the morning, or during your afternoon nap, and they come in at night just as you're falling asleep. It's imperative that they compare your pulse rates during your course of treatment.

We know now that pulse rate is not related merely to illness, but also to health. Sickness is indicated by a too rapid pulse, or one that's not beating rhythmically. Health is indicated by one's pulse-rate response to stress.

Your pulse is as singular as your signature or your fingerprint. It has a characteristic wave form. The wave may have a sharp peak, or be relatively flat. It might have subpeaks. It beats with a certain rhythmicity peculiar to your system. So distinctive is each pulse that a nurse in a ward filled with patients she had attended for some time could be blindfolded, led through shuffled beds and not only identify each patient from his pulse, but tell whether the patient was doing well or poorly that day.

With five minutes' training, you can learn to interpret your own well-being by taking your pulse. You can also note the difference in your emotional state from day to day. If you're excited, your pulse races. When you're calm and tranquil, your pulse reflects that rhythm. In a sense, the pulse is an aspect of your countenance.

Your normal pulse rate may be extremely fast or extremely slow compared to the norms—and yet be normal for you. You could have a pulse rate of ninety beats a minute while seated and yet be in better condition than someone with a normal rate of forty-five beats a minute.

YOUR PULSE RATE
GUIDES YOUR PROGRAM

However it beats at rest, it's your pulse rate during exercise that enables you to structure your fitness program exactly to your requirements. Your pulse rate is your individualized guide to fitness.

This program applies equally to men and women. The only persons who shouldn't attempt it are those whose doctors have forbidden exertion, or who fail the pulse test you'll be taking later on. Beyond that, the program is open regardless of age or physical condition. Those who are in the worst shape, in fact, will show the most dramatic and rapid improvement. If you haven't exercised once in the last twenty years, you are nonetheless just two hours away from good physical condition, relative to the condition you were in when you began. At the end of twelve hours, you'll be in excellent shape by any standards. You'll look and feel younger. Your waist will be thinner, your hips and thighs firmer. And you'll be permanently rid of many pounds of fat.

Those hours represent the cumulative time of three bouts of exercise a week of ten minutes each, during three courses of eight weeks each. You can do more if you wish. But the data say that you don't get much more good out of exercising every day than you do from exercising every other day. This is one program that discourages overzealousness.

The only price you pay for years of neglect is that it takes you a little longer to come back and you have a little further to go. You've already paid the price of low performance and a poor state of health for all the time you were out of shape. There are no further penalties, such as hard exercise.

The least little thing you do will measurably improve you. Consider the accountant who spends a solid month at his desk prior to the April 15th deadline for filing personal income tax. If he's been totally without exercise, his condition will be only twenty percent of what it was when the month began. But half an hour of activity that wouldn't normally be considered exercise—running errands or shopping—would restore twenty percent of the fitness he's lost. The first thirty feet of walking by a man who's recovering from surgery or been bedridden for several weeks will have a marked effect on his system. When your fitness is low, the least bit more of activity of any kind will change your strength, your muscular and cardio-respiratory endurance, help solidify your bones and resurrect your circulatory vessels.

THE JOYS OF PULSE-RATED EXERCISE

The maximum level of trainability for any man or woman is when he or she starts training at the age of ten and trains ever thereafter without getting sick. No one ever does that. All of us can only approach our potential. None of us ever reaches it. If you are fifty and you haven't worked out for twenty years, you can never get to the level of condition you would have achieved had you continued to play the tennis you played in college. If you had wanted to be the best possible sixty-year-old, the time to start was when you were ten. But you can start at fifty, having sloughed off since you were twenty, and be an astonishingly splendid sixty. You'll be in better shape than you were at fifty—even forty.

Actually, you may not be in such bad shape as you thought you were. If you've been climbing stairs or hauling heavy bags of groceries or polishing your car or even swinging a baby, you probably don't have far to go to be in decent shape.

There's no reason not to be in shape. It's so easy. It takes so little time. The response you get from the slightest amount of exercise is so great. You're immediately rewarded with a feeling of increased well-being. With exercise, you're livelier longer. The period during which you're half dead is reduced. And you reduce the prospects of premature death.

We'll start you with what you can do, no matter how little that is. Each day, you'll do just a little more, but so little that you'll scarcely notice. This all but infinitesimal increase is known as "overload." It's the foundation of pulse-rated exercise, and the key to its success.

Fitness is determined by what you do twenty-four hours a day, how you live, work, sit, walk, think, eat and sleep. Its purpose is to help you enjoy life, not to punish you or make you feel guilty. Life has enough burdens and prohibitions without adding to them. Just as you can become temporarily ill when you stop smoking, you can add to your deteriorative state by feeling anxious and guilty about skipping an exercise session, or by forcing yourself to do something you don't really enjoy doing.

This is not a young athlete's program. It's for the individual—man or woman—who wants a substantial reserve of fitness. It dispels late-day drag, makes physical recreation more enjoyable, gives you a sense of muscle tone, self-awareness and readiness, makes you more comfortable and secure because you know that if there's an emergency, you're better able to handle it. If you have to change a tire in the rain, you can do it without exhausting yourself. You can play an extra few sets of tennis with ease. You can stay up late when you have to. You can work an occasional eighteen-hour day and not need a week to recover. One not unimportant dividend is that you'll be a better lover.

I repeat: I hate formalized, rigid, punitive exercise. I hate it all the more now that I have the science to support my instinctive knowledge that it simply isn't necessary.

II

Fifteen Fitness Myths

Let's first dispense with the cant and misinformation that pervades the cult of fitness. If you're going to get yourself in shape, you'll want accurate, scientific guidelines, not the collection of old wives' tales that govern most people's exercise. When you see how wrong these accepted "principles" are, then perhaps you'll be ready to believe that fitness really is a piece of cake.

MYTH: NEVER DRINK WHILE EXERCISING

That couldn't be more wrong, You shouldn't even wait until you're thirsty. If you feel you're losing water, you should immediately replace it. And if you intend to exercise first thing in the morning, you should drink a glass of water before you start.

The body cells depend on circulation in order to get the energy they need, and to get rid of their waste products. When you become dehydrated, the fluids that bathe the cells diminish. The cells can't function properly until the fluid is restored. When that happens, your muscles can't keep up the work they're doing, and your heart receives an added strain. Part of the fluid you've lost is blood fluid. This means that the heart has to pump that many more times to recirculate the diminished supply of blood.

MYTH: SUGAR TAKEN BEFORE EXERCISE RAISES THE ENERGY LEVEL

Sugar ingested before a contest or workout can do more harm than good. Even preparations like honey and lemon juice are counterproductive. We've found by physiological studies that sweets can trigger an insulin reaction. The effect is to drive the body's sugar into the storage organs.

The only time you need to eat sugar to replace the amount that has been depleted is after an hour and a half of steady exercise, such as a marathon race or a golf or tennis match. Extra sugar never gives extra energy.

MYTH: AVOID CERTAIN FOODS BEFORE ACTIVITY

Extensive tests at UCLA's Human Performance Laboratory have yet to prove that the kind of food you eat makes the slightest difference in your performance or well-being. We combed the literature on this subject, picked out every food on the forbidden list and offered the food free to campus athletes. Heavy foods, gas-producing foods, spicy foods—we included them all. Neither on the playing field nor in the laboratory could players or researchers distinguish any difference. Nor did any of the players become sick from the "forbidden" foods.

MYTH: DON'T EAT BEFORE SWIMMING

How this one got started we'll never know. There's neither history nor science to support it. Cramps have never caused drowning. People who have supposedly drowned from cramps probably had heart attacks.

The theory against eating before swimming is that it draws the blood into your intestine; when you start exercising, according to this notion, the heart is unduly strained because muscles need blood, too. The fact is that once you start exercising, the circulation to the intestine shuts down and the blood goes to the muscles.

The most you might get if you exercise after eating is a stitch in the side. But cramps don't seem to be related to food at all. I knew one young American swimmer who ate a hamburger with onions and mustard, and four candy bars, and drank a Coke, just before a 1968 Olympics race, then broke her own world's record.

This isn't to suggest that you should eat a Thanksgiving dinner before swimming in a race. Any violent activity after a meal will cause nausea. But you can certainly paddle around a warm pool to your heart's content.

MYTH: USE SALT TABLETS TO PREVENT FATIGUE

Never. Salt tablets can be worse than no salt at all.

It's true that when you perspire copiously, you'll get muscle cramps unless you replace the salt. But a salt tablet is a solid piece of brine, and a solid piece of brine resting on the mucous membrane of the stomach can cause nausea and vomiting.

If you know you're going to perspire during a workout or contest, you can take a little extra salt with your food before hand. During the contest you can take some salt with water, or salt a piece of fruit. It's even a good idea to have some salt after your activity. But don't overdo it. Be sure you're only restoring salt that you've lost by sweating. The body can't store salt. If you overdo it, you may actually induce the cramps and muscular weakness you were trying to avoid. The fluids from the cells in your body will be drawn into the bloodstream and the digestive tract in order to dilute the salt so that it can be more easily excreted from the body. Just as you dry out meats to preserve them by soaking them in salt, so you've dried out the tissues of the body by overdoing the salt intake.

MYTH: EXTRA PROTEIN
MAKES YOU STRONG

So many athletes believe this, and so many food-supplement salespersons happily encourage them in their belief. Extra protein is a waste of money.

The body has tremendous reserves. It can make tremendous adaptations. The idea that you have to eat specified foods in specified amounts every day in order to maintain performance is unsound. I once did an experiment on the effects of starvation on work capacity. Three colleagues and I starved ourselves for four days and nights. We took nothing but water, not even chewing gum. I was a student at the time, at Springfield College, Massachusetts. Each day I went to classes, which included three physical-education activities. I even worked out with the wrestling team. I was surprised to find that after the third day, I wasn't all that hungry. The only time I'd crave food was when I'd pass a bakery or a hamburger stand. Several years later, in another experiment at the Harvard Fatigue Laboratory, we went without protein for a month. It wasn't until the end of the month that a deficiency in blood vitamin B showed up. Let me hastily add that my experiments didn't validate starvation as a good way to lose weight. Physiologists must be willing to punish themselves—to observe the effects of centrifugal force on their bodies, to see what freezing does to them, to start an experiment knowing they'll faint. That's their business. But they don't do it for kicks. The average person has no business starving himself to lose weight. When he does, there are consequences. Those experiments proved that the body has such large reserves of protein and fat that it doesn't need food supplements. They also proved what happens when you starve yourself for a prolonged period. I was sick as a dog afterward. For a month, my bowels didn't work properly, and I was weaker than I should have been.

When we're active, our body uses its own fat and carbohydrate for fuel. A diet that includes animal and vegetable protein supplies all the body needs to replenish its stores. There is no superdiet for superperformance. We've tried giving gelatin powder to athletes, on the assumption that it was high-protein, quick-energy magic. Our first studies showed that performance improved. But almost anything you take on the assumption that it will help *will* help. When more careful controls were applied, we learned that the only effect had been psychological.

The concept of the wide-variety diet, which we'll explore farther on, emerged from the futile search for a diet that would pay off. You need every kind of food. Avoiding any kind of food is just as wrong as ingesting food supplements.

MYTH: SLEEP EXTRA HOURS BEFORE A CONTEST, OR WHEN YOU'RE VERY TIRED

You can't store sleep. You can't catch up on sleep, either. If you try by sleeping twelve hours, you'll be worse off than if you got eight. Bed rest does not give you energy after eight hours, nine at most. A friend of mine refuses to believe that. "I know my body," she insists, "and I *know* that I benefit from twelve hours of sleep after several days with too little sleep. I get up feeling better." If she got up after nine hours, she would feel better yet. The further slight gain she may get in terms of repair and renewal is more than canceled out by her de-adaptation to increased activity. She becomes unfit.

Bed rest has a severe deconditioning effect. All the body processes slow down. After six hours, the heartbeat gets down to its basal rate. The metabolism lowers. Circulation becomes sluggish. The muscles become flaccid. The whole body begins to lose its tone. We've calculated that a person who's been inactive for three days has lost five percent of his strength. Remaining in bed for half a day diminishes the amount of time you can be active; thus the longer you remain in bed beyond a maximum of nine hours, the weaker you become.

Lying in bed in a relaxed state, incidentally, is almost as restful as sleeping. You get plenty of recovery. Rather than remaining in bed beyond eight hours because you haven't slept for worrying that

you wouldn't, get out of bed—and promise yourself to relax the next time you can't get to sleep.

MYTH: WORK UP A SWEAT BEFORE A CONTEST

You'd be better off taking a cold shower.

I know a runner who sits in the stands with his
girl friend eating watermelon until they call his
race. Then he goes onto the track and usually wins.
He may only be trying to psych his opponents. On
the other hand, he may be up-to-date on what
we've learned about warmups. In many cases, they're
counterproductive.

If you intend to go from absolute rest to all-out
exertion in a few seconds, this could cause failure
in circulation to the heart, which might be dangerous if your heart is weak. But if all you're going to
do is step up your activities gradually and play a
game that's not strenuous, then working up a
sweat is useless and could actually be disadvantageous if your activity is an endurance event. Warmups are okay for sprinters who want to practice
their starts. Any *skill* warmup, as distinguished from
a sweat warmup, is okay. But distance runners are
going to need all the energy they have, and they're
going to need to stay cool for as long as they can.
When the sweat starts dripping, they're finished.
"He left his race in his sweat suit" is a popular saying among runners. Nonetheless, they persist in
warming up in their sweat suits. That's got to hurt
their performance. We know that runners who stay

cool the longest perform the best. We once had a group of high-school runners stand in cold showers for ten minutes before they ran. To a man, they either matched their best performance or beat it. And they felt better after their race.

There are two reasons why prolonged warmups and working up a sweat are counterproductive: they deplete nutritional stores, and the body heat they create saps energy needed for the event. There's a lesson here for anyone embarking on a fitness program.

MYTH: SWEATING GETS YOU IN SHAPE

I know a tennis pro in Marina del Rey who wore a warmup suit while giving lessons, and got into the habit of wearing it during matches in order to lose weight. He started losing a lot of matches he should have won, to opponents he had previously beaten. Another man I know wore a rubber jacket over his sweat suit. He ran before he played tennis. Then he played vigorous tennis, mopping himself with a towel so he could see. "Jim, you're getting out of shape," I told him. "All you're conditioning yourself for is heat acclimatization. When you get such body heat, you can't work hard enough to get into good condition. Play cool and you can work harder, and thereby get into better condition for tennis."

Rubberized suits may acclimatize you to heat—which is a good idea if you intend to play tennis in the tropics or fight in the desert—but they do absolutely nothing else for you, and they can very well endanger your life.

The basic rule of working out is to avoid dripping sweat whenever possible. It takes energy to lose heat. This energy comes from the activity of your sweat glands; millions of them lying just under your skin use metabolic energy to secrete sweat. This energy is drained from the total energy you have at your command to do the work of your body. Your muscles have to share in this energy in order to function properly. If a disproportionate share of that energy is used to secrete sweat, then there isn't enough left for your other bodily functions. The amount of work you can do lessens when sweat glands use energy. When exhausted, they stop secreting, and you're in peril of a heat stroke.

The second loss of energy when you overheat is in your cardiovascular system. When the skin gets hot, the peripheral vessels leading to the skin open. The big part of your blood supply rushes to the surface of your body. This deprives the muscles of the blood they need. The heart tries to make up for the loss by pumping harder. The load becomes so great that if it's maintained for a prolonged period you could collapse, and conceivably die. Inducing sweat is dangerous and it makes no contribution to fitness.

The best clothing for hot-weather exercise is a naked skin. If you're exercising indoors, your underwear is just fine. If you're working in the garden, jogging, or playing tennis or golf, your clothing should be lightweight and light in color. The difference between a dark shirt and a light shirt can mean the difference between comfort and discomfort.

There is no danger in being comfortably cool while you're working hard. It's an absolute disadvantage to be uncomfortably warm. It's even disadvantageous when sleeping. Not long ago, the mother of a friend of mine was sliding downhill fast for no apparent reason. She was active. Her diet was okay. She'd been to the doctor; he'd found nothing wrong with her. It was just at this time that I happened to be studying the effects of heat storage on energy. So I asked her if, by chance, she was using an electric blanket. Yes, she said, as a matter of fact, she'd just received one for Christmas. So I asked her to check the setting. It turned out that she had been using the blanket like an electric heating pad, and had been bathed in sweat all night. I advised her to turn the blanket down to a low setting that took the chill off the bed but didn't overheat her. Her energy bounded back immediately.

Sweating *does* make the heart work harder, which is an objective of a fitness workout, but it does so in a hazardous manner. In exercise, you can control the pumping of your heart simply by stopping what you're doing. But when you overload your heart by overheating your body, there's no way you can stop the process except by jumping into some ice water.

Sweating *does* burn calories, but it's a dangerous way to reduce. You could have the best figure in the morgue. That's a remote possibility, but why take a chance?

The basic point to remember is this: You have only so much energy available. It takes a lot of energy to lose heat. If you use your energy this way, you won't have the energy you need to accomplish the task that's making you hot. Off with the sweat suits! Away with rubberized garments!

MYTH: PUT ON A SWEATER AFTER EXERCISE

This one is Grandmother's favorite. It's nonsense, too. There is no point in prolonging heat by encasing it in a garment. As to the notion that you're courting a cold, it's conceivable that some part of your body such as your neck might get stiff, but you don't catch cold by changing temperature. I've sat for hours in a cold chamber with other human guinea pigs. We were studying how the body regulates temperature. We shivered a lot but never caught cold. We didn't develop stiff necks either.

After sweaty exercise, help your body to recover its normal state by leaving off your sweater. When you no longer feel hot and your sweating has subsided, put on your sweater to keep from getting chilly. You'll be more comfortable not staying overheated so long.

MYTH: TAKE A COLD SHOWER AFTER A HOT ONE IN ORDER TO CLOSE YOUR PORES

Totally unnecessary. A cool shower after a warm one may feel good, but a really cold one should be avoided even if you're a masochist and enjoy it. Not only do you do yourself no good by subjecting yourself to this torture, you could be endangering your life. My old friend George Folsey, a Hollywood film photographer, loved to finish off with a cold shower. He couldn't understand why he got a pain in his chest. What he had done was induce an attack of angina. The cold water caused a constriction of the vessels in his heart as well as in his skin. Vessels aren't pores. Pores don't have to be "closed."

MYTH: NEVER EXERCISE IN THE HOT NOON SUN

As Noel Coward put it in a song, only "mad dogs and Englishmen" go out in the noonday sun. Actually, it's the safest time to exercise on a sunny day. With the sun overhead, all you need to shield yourself is a hat. In midmorning or midafternoon, however, there is no way to shield your body from direct exposure to the sun's rays coming in at an angle.

MYTH: AVOID SEX BEFORE ATHLETICS

The popular notion that abstinence somehow stores strength has no scientific foundation. Athletes are subject to all kinds of constraints. The more constraints you remove from them, the better they perform. Athletes seem to do better after sexual intercourse, even when they have intercourse the morning of a competition. Enlightened coaches encourage players to bring their mates along with them.

MYTH: WOMEN WHO TRAIN LOSE FEMININITY

To the contrary. They become more feminine, more sexy, and increase their animal vitality. They are more lithe, they move with greater strength, and they develop the athlete's sense of relaxation—an air of languor under which lies a supply of power waiting to be used.

Women who lift weights and do gymnastic exercises develop firm muscles, but because of their thicker subcutaneous layer of fat they don't form bulges the way men do. The body retains its female contours. Muscular development of the chest enhances the breast line. The hips and thighs, the main trouble spots for women, are slimmed by exercise.

MYTH: BIG MUSCLES MAKE
YOU STRONGER

We all believed that twenty years ago. Today we know that you can get stronger without enlarging your muscles, that you can enlarge your muscles without much increase in strength, and that big muscles might not have been such a good idea in the first place.

It does not necessarily follow that big muscles are strong muscles, that strong muscles are better-performing muscles and that better-performing muscles are healthier muscles. Except for those who need massive bodies to put against heavy loads, champions accept the fact today that they should keep their muscles small. That information, alas, has not filtered down to our fitness palaces. These establishments are still promulgating a body-beautiful notion that is out of date and discredited.

In the early 1900s, Dr. Dudley Sargent of Harvard University began to modify the calisthenic exercises and gymnastics that had emerged from Sweden and Germany. Both systems had originated on the farms; both had been designed to make the body look better. Dr. Sargent promoted the notion of the ideal American man and woman. In his laboratory, he had taken thousands of measurements of athletes, using tape measures, calipers and stadiometers. He developed detailed charts showing what the girth of arms, waists, chests and legs should be. He devised whole systems of exercises that would change body measurements to conform to his standards.

The effort made to achieve an ideal physique did cause some improvement in the individual's fitness. But fitness wasn't the goal. The goal was to make an ideal physique. The delusion persists today. Look into any body-building gym or health club or reducing salon; you'll find statues of Greek gods and goddesses, and pictures of improbable men and women. The people who patronize these establishments want to make their bodies conform. No deference is shown to individual differences. Nor is any consideration given to what's happening inside the body. It doesn't matter that the individual may be approaching heart disease or be incapable of relaxing. If he looks well, he's fit. Hollywood men look great. They have slim waists and suntans. They have also got ulcers.

Looking great is desirable. It may be a byproduct of a good fitness program. But it's not the acid test of fitness, and it shouldn't be the primary objective of a fitness program. The major objective should be to develop a high-quality body possessed of vigor and the capacity to resist stress and strain.

Ironically, this popular, Tarzan-like symbol of fitness for men, a large chest, shoulders and arms, can be a detriment to performance. Hypertrophy—increase in muscle mass—means an extra weight to carry around and an impairment of movement. In a sense, it's like being obese; instead of hypertrophy of fat cells, you develop hypertrophy of muscle cells.

But it's the misleading objective put into the individual's mind that causes the most trouble. The person who perceives his goal to be unattainable winds up doing nothing at all. So long as these false images of fitness persist in the public mind, most people will be discouraged from embarking on a genuine fitness program. If exercise means that you've got to go down to some gym and spend money to engage in an hour of heavy, torturous manual labor in order to struggle toward nonattainable goals, you're going to be turned off. Small wonder that most people don't exercise.

We live life with more than enough constraints and regulations. To add false goals, needless exercise, strict regimens, sexual abstinence and dietary regulations that serve no purpose is an inhuman—and biologically unnecessary—demand.

What I'm against is the kind of rigid discipline which says that every morning at six o'clock you've got to fling open the windows, gulp ten breaths of fresh air, do your daily dozen and take an ice-cold shower, then have a breakfast of seaweed and vitamin pills. It's all unnecessary for good health, and it *may* do more harm than good.

This isn't to say that breathing fresh air isn't okay, or that taking exercise isn't beneficial, or that eating wholesome food is contraindicated. It's to say that you don't need to force yourself into a life style that is actually a strain. Most people are already overburdened with too many requirements. They have to be up at a fixed time, get to work at a fixed time, get their work done at a certain rate, earn a certain amount of money. These requirements can be so much of a strain that they're unhealthful. To impose on top of them obligations that really aren't necessary is folly.

A hostess isn't happy unless her guests are uncomfortably stuffed. We apply the same perverse reasoning to exercise. It's not exercise unless we're uncomfortable.

THE TYRANNY OF FITNESS TEACHERS

I regret to say so, but many leaders of physical exercise aren't satisfied unless their charges' tongues are hanging out at the end of a workout. These drillmasters suffer from an affliction I call ergomania—a craze for work. They possess an almost obnoxious enthusiasm for exercise. They don't think that exercise is any benefit unless you're sweating —or bleeding, if possible.

William Sheldon of Yale divides body types into mesomorphs, ectomorphs and endomorphs. Mesomorphs are the heavily muscled, heavy-boned, square, stocky individuals. They love strenuous physical activity and body contact. They like to perspire and they don't mind bleeding. They thrive on hard competition. The best time of their lives is when they've finished a workout and get into the shower. They probably finish off with a cold shower. This is the type of individual who usually becomes a physical-training director. They have no sympathy for ectomorphs and endomorphs.

Ectomorphs are the thin, frail, nervous type. By nature, they can't stand still. By the time they come to a gym class, they may already have had enough physical activity for the day. Nonetheless, they'll cooperate with the physical director because they're active by nature. They're easily driven to exhaustion.

Endomorphs hate exercise and leaders of exercise. They're the round, soft, flabby people who love ease and comfort. They resist the physical director's superenergy. They hide in dark corners when it's time to choose up for foot races. They're the physical director's favorite target. The director wants to change the endomorph into his own image. He wants his softness to be hardness, his love of Athenian comfort to transfer to affection for Spartan discomfort.

Most of the books on exercise are written by mesomorphs with endomorphs as their targets.

The worst sin of all is when physical-training instructors use exercise as a punitive device. In many high schools, if a student is out of line he is made to do a certain number of pushups or run so many laps around a track. Exhaustive exercise is thought to be some kind of character builder. In the police academies, it's used as a screening device to weed out candidates with weak "character." In punitive programs, the goal of the drill instructor is to make the students stiff and sore. The theory is that they haven't been sufficiently worked until the point of pain is reached. This leads the unsuspecting pupils to believe that self-punishment is a part of exercise. The disease spreads over into community fitness programs. I meet individuals in parks and playgrounds who believe that without pain there is no progress—like Gene Tunney, who would run in the cold at night until he felt he could go no farther, and then keep on running.

Such programs produce discouragement, injury and, occasionally, death. It's all so needless.

The images of what it takes to be a champion have been applied to what it takes to be fit—veins about to pop, gasping for air, pain. It's not only a bad image for fitness, it may be bad for champions. One of my students at UCLA was James McAlister, who in addition to being a superb football player is a world-class broad jumper. The night before an important track meet, he went nightclubbing with some old friends who were competing against him in the same meet. "I got two things off," he told me on his return. "I saw my old buddies, and I broke my record."

Coaches are discovering that many of the constraints they've been putting on athletes aren't necessary and just add to the noxious burden of an athlete's training. I've been a coach, I've made these mistakes. It isn't necessary to "toe the line" or "snap to." Training tables, bed checks, the separation of college athletes from other students in special dorms—these liken the athlete to a circus animal. Senseless training rules and regulations force the coach to become an animal trainer, whipping his athletes into submission. The best athletic performances come from players who feel "on their own" to get themselves ready for their games. Certainly, the good coach gives strong directions and makes final decisions. But he doesn't burden his players with unreasonable injunctions. He knows his physiology of exercise. He will not prohibit milk "because it cuts the wind." (He knows it doesn't.) Diet isn't all that important. Neither is a full night's sleep. We've learned a great deal since Eleanor Holm was kicked off the U.S. Olympic swimming team for drinking a glass of champagne aboard ship. There are lessons galore for fitness.

Jim McAlister knows it's not necessary to be a Spartan to be a champion. Exhaustion and regimentation are no part of his regimen. They shouldn't be part of yours.

III

Fit for What?

Let's suppose you've established an amenable life style. You have a comfortable home that meets your social and psychological needs. Your children are either in college or preparing to go. Your investments exceed your indebtedness, and you're well insured. On top of that, you've got a little money in the bank, and you're working at a level that comfortably maintains this status. How much better off would you be if you worked twice as hard? The chances are that you wouldn't be all that much better off—and you might conceivably be worse. The extra work would subtract from the time you have to enjoy yourself. And it might make you sick.

The trap of rising expectations is as great a potential snare for the person who wants to be fit as it is for the one who wants to be rich. If getting more stimulates your need for still more, you'll never be satisfied. The secret of happiness is a goal you can achieve. When a woman determines to model herself on a beauty out of *Vogue,* she has charted a course to despair. The way to achieve fitness is to be delighted with anything that takes you from where you are right now to being a little better.

A flat belly looks great. With a tremendous amount of effort, you can develop the kind of rock-hard abdomen that has the gymnast's groove down the center. If you're willing to work that much each day to look that great, fine. But you don't really need a belly that's as hard as a rock to be fit. You can have a more than adequate, pleasing abdomen with a minimum amount of exercise.

If you want to be fit enough to do a hundred handstand pushups, fine. But how much more fit does it make you for the real requirements of your life? The hundred-handstand-pushup man is really not that much more healthy in terms of preventing deterioration, and not that much more fit for ordinary emergencies, than he would be with a much less rigorous program.

Suppose you're a golfer. Golf requires power. The movement is explosive. It requires muscular strength. If your strength is deficient, then your ability to develop power is limited. If we put you on a weight training program to develop muscular strength, your power will improve, and so will your game. But there is a certain point beyond which power does no further good. If you continue to develop your strength, you won't be able to put it to advantage. You're wasting time and energy. You'd be much better off if you devoted time and energy to sharpening your game.

We need a certain amount of muscle strength and endurance and circulo-respiratory endurance in order to live well and carry out our daily activities effectively and without fatigue. But to train our-selves to very high levels would give us very little more health and fitness for everyday living than we can achieve in a thirty-minutes-a-week pulse-rated exercise program. In those thirty minutes, as you'll soon see, you'll exercise all the muscles that need exercise, to just the right degree.

A SINGLE ACTIVITY WON'T DO

Most people who embark on a fitness program look for the one activity that will do everything for them. Weight lifters feel they can get everything they're ever going to need from weight lifting. The tennis player thinks that tennis is the complete sport. Joggers assume that all good things will happen so long as they keep jogging. Conclusions or premises like these are predictive of failure in fitness pro-grams. The jogger, for example, can run a mile in eight minutes every day for a year. At the end of the year, he will be in worse shape than he was at the end of the second month. For the first two months, running a mile would improve his condi-tion. But if he continues to run the mile in exactly the same way, he will adapt to that demand, his responses will diminish and he will begin to "de-condition." We'll get into that phenomenon farther on.

Each different type of physical load has its specific conditioning effect, period. Sprint runs do not build endurance for distance runs. Swimming does not develop muscular strength. Weight lifting does not improve cardiovascular condition. Although exercise in any form is beneficial, no one exercise develops general fitness. Several types of exercise are necessary for all-around development.

The concept of fitness is implicit in the word. Fit for what?

Not long ago, I was asked by the Los Angeles Police Academy to set up a fitness program for its cadets. In reviewing past and present programs, I discovered a pattern. The present physical-training instructor was a prizefighter. He had all the cadets punching bags, skipping rope and sparring with one another. The previous instructor had been a track man. His fitness program resembled a track meet. The academy was at the mercy of the person it hired. No consideration had been given to what kinds of fitness requirements police work entailed. I arranged to have one of my investigators accompany various policemen on their rounds to make a study of their duties. On the basis of his findings, we concluded that the police had to be fit for short bursts of activity. When they chased a subject, if they didn't catch him in the first fifty yards, they'd find some other way to go after him. The police have to pay for their own uniforms, as well as repairs to them; if it meant climbing over a fence to apprehend a suspect, they figured the hell with it. The suspects they caught were surprisingly strong; if the suspect was a homosexual, he was probably a body builder. We had always thought of the policeman as the strong man and the criminal as the weak man, but now our image began to change. We went into prisons and tested the strength of criminals, on the assumption that the policemen should be at least as strong as their adversaries. Out of this study we defined with greater accuracy the fitness needs of the policemen, and described a different program. Instead of the five-mile runs that are a fixture of most police academy programs, we prescribed intervals of fifty-yard dashes. Instead of punching bags we used weight training. We stepped up hand-to-hand combat drills, and restraint procedures.

ASK YOURSELF WHO YOU ARE

Before you can set out a fitness program, you must first define who you are. My collaborator, Leonard Gross, has a program for a writer, husband, father, skier and tennis player. If we had written a program for the writer, husband and father, he would have had a completely different program. There would have been no demands for extremes in performance. By adding tennis and skiing, we had to provide for a high degree of muscle and circulo-respiratory endurance.

The objective is to be fit for what you are. If you're not a tennis player or a skier, you really don't need the level of fitness a tennis player or a skier requires.

Training for fitness falls exactly between physical therapy at one end of the scale and athletic performance at the other. The same basic principles apply—but in an entirely different way.

In therapy, the problem is deterioration of muscle. So the first objective is to get the muscle bigger, in order to have sufficient tissue. You can't make a muscle stronger if there's not sufficient tissue to strengthen. To do that, patients must be encouraged to extend their effort until they unconsciously substitute other muscles in an effort to achieve their objectives. The point of therapy is to get them to use muscles that have been dormant. When they start using the rest of their bodies to help lift a leg, instead of just using the leg muscle, then they're on their way back to normal.

In athletics, the objective is to increase athletes' tolerance to that extra second or two of effort that can make them champions. It's that peak effort which adds the fraction they need for better performance.

Neither situation applies in physical-fitness training. Not only should you not feel pushed, you shouldn't even feel uncomfortable.

Organic fitness is basic to all activities. It's not training for an athletic event, but it must precede training for that event. Without organic fitness, you aren't ready for the training. People who play three fast sets of tennis every Sunday morning and do nothing else during the week are apt to injure themselves. But if they're maintaining a comfortable reserve of fitness, they're prepared for their Sunday session.

I would never train athletes the way I train people to stay fit; when you start athletic training, it's presumed you're in good physical condition. I wouldn't prescribe therapeutic exercise for healthy persons; it would be far below their needs. I wouldn't prescribe a fitness program for a patient who is injured or ill; you don't start such a program until your rehabilitation is complete.

If you aren't an athlete and you're not a patient recovering from an illness, you need a fitness program. Your needs are different from theirs. Your program should be, too.

FITNESS ISN'T HEALTH

Health, fitness and performance are three separate and poorly correlated phenomena.

Health is generally defined as the freedom from disease.

Fitness strictly relates to your ability to meet the demands of your environment.

Performance is how well you accomplish a task.

You can be healthy without being fit. You can be in poor health and perform superbly. Sick athletes break records all the time. Every Olympic competition is populated by athletes with colds, fevers, infections and diarrhea. They invariably compete, and perform to their level.

The idea that sports make you healthy is a shibboleth. Sports can actually hurt you. They're not unhealthy *per se,* but they can be.

You don't have to be fit to be healthy. If health is defined as lack of disease, then fitness is not health. Only when your definition of health includes functional wellness—meaning the ability to cope with your environment—do health, fitness and performance coincide.

I was at a faculty picnic a few years back, swimming with a colleague of mine, John Sellwood. He was dying of lung cancer. One lung had been removed; the other was infected. He was to go into the hospital the next day. Both of us had been college swimmers. We'd been swimming for a while when he said, "I'll race you fifty yards."

"You've already given me my handicap," I said, and I thought it gave me an unfair advantage. We started off even. I didn't deliberately let him beat me, but he did. The next day he entered the hospital, and a month later he was dead. I can think of no better illustration of the lack of correlation between health and performance.

Fitness means the development of components —muscular strength, muscular endurance, cardiovascular endurance and flexibility.

Suppose I go to a gym and develop all these components? Am I going to swim or ski or play basketball better? Probably not. Supposing I just played basketball or skied or swam?

If my objective is to play a sport better, I would do better to play that sport. If I go swimming, play basketball or ski, I improve my performance in that sport—but it may make only a negligible contribution to my general muscular and cardio-respiratory fitness.

We have a name for this phenomenon in physiology. It's called *specificity*. It means that if you want to train for an event, you practice that event, or exercise in a manner that simulates its requirements. For those who enjoy a sport, I'll offer some supplementary suggestions later on about how you can improve your performance. But right now our task is to get you in shape for everyday life, so that you'll look younger and feel better and not sag at the end of the day.

GETTING IN SHAPE TO GET IN SHAPE

Why do people who have avoided exercise for so long start to exercise?

One day, you find you're not in charge of your life any more. You've been overcome by your job, your family responsibilities, the need to pay your bills. On that particular day, you've noticed while shaving or making up your face that your shoulders, which were once muscular and well set, are now bony and sagging. Everything in your body has seemed to move down to the center of your frame. One of your closest friends has just died of a heart attack. Or you've gone outside to climb a hill or romp with your children, have a catch or even play tennis, and within a few minutes you're breathless. From any or all of these signals, you've decided to do something about your condition.

If all you decide to do is use a flight of stairs in lieu of an elevator, it's going to do wonders.

Years ago, I made a series of faculty conditioning studies at three universities—Iowa, Harvard and Southern California. A month after the program was initiated, one of the professors came to me and confessed that he couldn't get interested in the program I had outlined for him. He abhorred calisthenics. "The only thing I did differently," he said, "was to climb a flight of stairs instead of taking the elevator." He paused. "I don't know how to explain it, but it made a world of difference."

I could see from his appearance that it had. But I couldn't understand from my knowledge of the physiology of exercise, as well as my work on muscles, heart and blood, why that one change had affected him physiologically. Before long, however, the same thing began occurring among others in the program. They too had eschewed the calisthenics. But they had made one small change in their daily patterns.

The results went up against all the theories I had been taught to that point. The basic theory was that hard exercise was necessary to maintain good physical condition. But here were numbers of persons showing dramatic changes just by altering one habit.

I questioned them all. It developed that persistence about the new habit had affected many habits. They smoked less, avoided junk food, slept better, drank with greater moderation. One increment in their lives had altered their philosophic view about personal maintenance.

If you make an investment in exercise, it makes you conscious of other reasonable health habits. You're not about to waste your investment.

IT'S THE PAST FOUR WEEKS
THAT COUNT

The body adjusts to the demands you put on it from day to day. Any exertion beyond a light effort is an overload—and will stimulate development. The effort can be mild, and still be stimulating.

If you have a job in which you regularly have to exert a heavy effort, you may be getting all the exertion you need to be fit. You don't need anything extra unless you're going to do something different; ditch digging won't make you fit for skiing.

The body also adjusts to the lack of demand that you put on it. If you diminish demand, your body will immediately register that fact. Each week, your body will reflect what you did—or didn't do—the previous week. Your heredity, medical profile and athletic habits are factors in your present condition, but what you have done—or not done—habitually in the last four weeks of your life is infinitely more important in determining what kind of shape you're in today.

Supposing you're a healthy person, you've been vigorously active all your life and there is no history of illness in your family. You're in famous shape. One day, you become involved in a matter so pressing that you're unable to leave your desk for a month. Each week of that month, your condition will deteriorate. By the end of the month, you will have lost eighty percent of the condition you had. On a scale of one hundred, you'll be

at twenty. Two weeks later if you still haven't en-
gaged in physical activity, you'll be at ten.

Supposing the contrary is true: you've avoided
exercise all your life. You can, within a month, raise
your level of conditioning from somewhere near
zero to eighty.

Some people don't want to be in good condition. Consciously or unconsciously, they've decided
that they prefer to be soft, flabby and weak. They
want to be nursed, or cared for. They want to avoid
responsibility. Or they want to be thought of as sensitive intellectual brains. Whatever the motivation,
these people "de-adapt" themselves, reducing all
physical demands on their body in order to achieve
the desired image of a small, weak, physically ineffective person. They train themselves to be frail.

If, however, you're the kind of person who is
naturally predisposed to physical activity but has
been deprived of it because of your job or the
pressures of living, your first step is to take a hard
look at your life style on the assumption that it's
literally killing you. If you want to live a normal
life span, you've got to become active.

My wife says, "I envy you. You bowl on Monday nights. You play golf on Thursday and Saturday
afternoon. You play tennis on Sunday morning and
Wednesday afternoon, and you're looking for someone to play with on Tuesdays and Fridays." I re-
ply, "It's not easy to preserve these moments for
yourself. No one is managing your life and saying,
'You must save time for exercise.' You have to decide yourself what you want to do with your time
and energy. If your schedule doesn't include things

you enjoy that are good for you, then it's up to you to readjust your life style."

HOW TO TURN YOUR LIFE AROUND

If you see yourself in such a bind, and that you're deteriorating in the process, then you'd better take a good look at your job, your life style and your domestic situation and do something about one or all of them. No employer or spouse has the right to deprive another person of his normal function and structure. If you let yourself get into the habit of bills and children and shopping, you've allowed yourself to be trapped. If you enjoy activities and can't do them, it's doubly frustrating. When, on top of all that, you're ashamed of what you see in your mirror, it's time to turn your life around and get some activities into your pattern. There are three steps to such a change that don't involve any exercise.

The first step is simply to accept the importance of physical activity. You can always find time to do the things you really want to do.

The second step is to schedule the activity in spite of everything else you have to do. It becomes one of the high-priority items of your life.

The third step is to work on your attitude to exercise.

There are at least fifteen excuses we can find not to exercise. It's contrary to our life style. No one else does it; if we did it, they'd ridicule us. We have motors now to do what muscles once had to do. Our physical facilities for exercise are too small and confining. We don't know enough about exercise. We don't have the skill. We've got something better to do when the chance to exercise arises. We've got something more pressing to do. We'll fall. We'll have a heart attack. We'll disgrace ourselves. We'll look terrible. It will tire us. It will make us sore. It will give us a headache or backache.

Occasionally, there's even medical argument against exercise. I know of one doctor, surely a philosophical determinist, who maintains that your heart is programmed for just so many heartbeats, and when you've used up the last one you die. It follows from this argument that an activity which speeds up the heart is to be avoided at all costs. Let's suppose the theory were true. It would make all the more sense to exercise, because the heartbeat of a well-conditioned person is slower by a good ten beats a minute at rest than it would be if he were out of shape.

We all know that our capacity to perform declines with age. But we must ask whether the decline is an inevitable result of age, or whether it's induced by the change in what we do. As we grow older, we perform less. The process becomes self-fulfilling. Our diminished effort further diminishes our ability to exert. It follows that if we were to increase our effort, we would increase our capacity to exert.

"I'M TOO OLD *NOT* TO EXERCISE"

Not long ago, the Los Angeles Public School System commissioned me to give a series of lectures on gerontology to classes of elderly people. The lectures were held in high schools, retirement homes and ballrooms. As many as five hundred people came each time. I not only lectured on exercise, I taught members of the audience to work their faces, necks, legs and arms while sitting in their chairs. They got a terrific kick out of the exercises, and apparently did them daily thereafter, because subsequent reports all indicated how much better they felt and how much the program had affected their lives. Some of the testimonials were from people in their nineties.

Most elderly people aren't like that, unfortunately. They feel they're getting enough exercise even though they're doing no exercise at all. The older they get, the more inclined they are to say that they're exercising enough. They accept age as an excuse for inactivity. They say, "I'm too old to exercise." They should say, "I'm too old *not* to exercise."

Most adults who engage in any exercise at all take it so easy and participate for such short periods that they hardly increase their heart or breathing rate. Only three out of every hundred Americans participate in an organized fitness program. Eighty-five percent of the public doesn't own any exercise equipment, not even a pair of sneakers. These people have a problem just as special as that of the patient on the mend or the athlete on a championship training program. The patient knows what he needs to recuperate. The athlete knows what he needs to be a winner. The person in between is really in limbo. He knows what he wants, but not what he needs.

What he wants is a more youthful appearance and the strength and stamina to go with it. What he needs is a reduction in excess body fat, an increase in muscle mass and tone and an improvement in circulo-respiratory endurance.

POSITIVE REINFORCEMENT

Studies in Veterans Administration hospitals have shown us that the first step in rehabilitation is to enlarge a person's concept of himself as an effective human being. One means is to enlarge his body. It's not so much the muscles he develops as it is the new feeling of muscle awareness that convinces him he's more effective. He feels the presence of himself the day he starts his program.

Behavioral science has taught us that good behavior is stimulated by positive reinforcement. There's plenty of reinforcement built into the conditioning process: feeling better is a terrific payoff. But you have to be certain that you'll receive encouragement from others if you're embarking on a program. Conversely, if it's your spouse who's starting out, *you* should be offering encouragement. I know many a woman who has nipped an exercise program in the bud simply by disparaging her husband the day he starts to work out. She'll suggest he looks ridiculous. She'll stare at his bouncing flab. Or she'll ignore him. If you want to erase a habit, you ignore it. If you want a habit to persist, you praise it. Every day that my wife gets on her stationary bicycle to have a workout, I say, "Good girl." One day I forgot. She said, "You didn't say 'Good girl.'" Years ago, when I owned a home with a pool, I asked my wife to tell me, when I got home from work, "Why don't you have a little swim, dear?" I knew I was getting my own words back, but it was still enough to get me into the pool.

A few years ago, the wife of a friend of mine came to me. "I can't get him to do anything," she complained. "He won't even walk the dog." I suggested that she praise her husband whenever he did the least little thing physical, even if it was to step outside for a breath of air. If he suggested they go window shopping, she should leap at the chance. "Make him feel good about doing it," I urged her. Now he's walking the dog.

The only way you'll stick to your program is if you find you enjoy it. So your objective should be to make your exercise as much fun as possible. At a minimum, you should try to get rid of the understandable bias you picked up against exercise in the military service or in school.

IGNORE THE "PRE-START PHENOMENON"

Past experience has conditioned us to the belief that any exertion will be uncomfortable, potentially injurious or a drudge. So we apply this preconditioned attitude to all exertion, whether valid or not. We actually feel ill at times, usually sick to the stomach.

The way you feel before exertion has no relation to how you'll perform. The opposite can be true. The worse you feel, the better you may perform. This is because your fear and anxiety have called forth a secretion of adrenaline, which strengthens muscular contractions. The nervousness that accompanies the flow is known as the "pre-start phenomenon." If you haven't got it, you feel more comfortable, but don't bet too much on your golf game. The days when you feel awful are often the days when you'll shoot your best game.

Mel Patton, who was the fastest human in the world when he ran for the University of Southern California, always vomited before his better races.

There is a difference between how you feel about approaching exercise and how you feel during exercise. You have to differentiate between this apprehension phenomenon and a true state of illness. If you do have an infection that is making you sick, then you should skip your exercise that day. But knowing about the pre-start phenomenon, you should be able to distinguish between illness and apprehension. Once you start the workout, the pre-start feeling disappears, and your perceptions of the exertion become extremely accurate.

Ergomaniacs who try to sell fitness to others not so afflicted kill off the whole idea of exercise. I know one man so dedicated that he exercises for thirty minutes every morning regardless of whether he is dead tired or has a fever. The morning that he misses his exercise will be the morning after his death. The point is that he's often doing himself more harm than good. He shouldn't be exercising when he's sick or overfatigued. He won't lose a thing by skipping a bout.

I don't exercise if I think something may be wrong with me. One day recently, I awakened with a strange, sickly feeling, something like the one I have when I've had too much to drink. But I'd had nothing the night before. The feeling persisted for a week, and in that week I didn't exercise. Whatever it was, the illness was taken care of naturally. I then resumed my program. In another week, I had regained my proper level of fitness.

In the week that I didn't exercise, I could see the consequences. My midsection turned soft. I had no feeling of tone. I felt mushy all through my system. Yet it didn't worry me that I had let my fitness slip.

If you've got a regular exercise routine and something happens to make you skip it, you shouldn't feel guilty. But it's terribly important to distinguish between lack of health and lack of inclination. The latter is entirely unrelated to your capacity to perform, and should be ignored. Conceivably, you're not well. Far more likely, you're experiencing the pre-start phenomenon.

You've got to psych yourself up for exercises. In *Visions of Eight,* David Wolper's film of the 1972 Olympics, there was a fragment on a giant Russian weight lifter who kept approaching his weight, only to shake his head and back off. Many times he approached it, looked at it, muttered to himself and walked away. Finally he ran to it, attempted to lift it and fell over backward. His experience is not unlike yours. You are saying to that weight, "I am going to lift you." And the weight is saying, "Oh, no, I'm too heavy. You better not lift me. I'm going to hurt you." Sometimes the weight psychs you out. It conquered the Olympian. It can conquer you in your bedroom.

I don't want you ever in that kind of situation. You're not trying to lift a certain load or race against the clock. Those aren't good objectives. There are days when you just can't meet them—and, besides, they don't tell you what's happening to you as a consequence of your effort. The proper objective is one that is consistent with how you feel or what kind of exertion is going to feel right for you.

BEWARE OF CRASH PROGRAMS

It's important that you don't get ambitious and try a crash program. Inevitably, you'll have to pick up the pieces. You'll probably give up your program altogether. It took you many years to get in the shape you're in. You can well afford a program that has you feeling and looking *somewhat* better almost immediately and a great deal better in a few months. Exercise should always be a happy experience, where you feel good at the end of every bout.

Unfortunately, we're in competition with programs that promise the stars. You'll lose a pound a day, seven pounds in a week, they tell you. What they *don't* tell you is that in order to do that you must starve. To demand that a person lose even two pounds a week is an inhuman request. It requires that you diet in a manner that almost surely results in illness. And almost surely, you'll gain back the pounds that you've lost.

We know from studies of behavioral science that people aren't going to make drastic changes in their habits and life style. The only exceptions are people who do things like joining an Israeli kibbutz. When a big-city banker voluntarily becomes a farm laborer, that's an extreme and unusual change. Most people can't do it. It's very easy to get a smoker to change his brand, but it's extremely difficult to persuade him to stop smoking. The chances are only one in three hundred that an alcoholic can be cured. In considering changes in your fitness habits, try to be realistic. To double your physical strength and endurance and bring you to par with a trained athlete requires a minimum of two hours a day of strenuous exertion. That's not a realistic goal; you haven't got the time, patience, inclination or need. You'll do extremely well with less.

YOU'RE NOT COMPETING WITH ANYONE

One day I was demonstrating my own workout to a friend of mine. "I can't do that," he muttered. I really laid into him. "Don't compare your needs to mine," I scolded. "When you're in the business of physical development and maintenance, you're out of the business of competition. You don't compete with anybody—least of all yourself."

You're not trying to lift more weight than someone else. This doesn't measure your fitness. You're not setting out to lift two hundred pounds or run a mile in six minutes. These are athletic objectives; *your* objectives aren't athletic. The word "athletic" means to defeat someone. There's no defeat in the fitness program.

Your attitude should be: This is my own program. I'm going to do it in the privacy of my home. No one else is going to know about it if I don't want them to. And it won't be like any other program in the world.

Exercise doesn't have to include activities you hate. For every person who loves to jog, there are probably ten thousand who hate it. Out there looking ridiculous in unflattering clothes with everyone staring at you—who needs it?

Physical exercise is a sensuous activity. When you move, you should have the feeling of grace and rhythm. Your stretch should be languorous. Your stride should be pleasant. When you're working against a stopwatch instead of your own natural rhythm, it's then that exercise becomes a drudgery. Exercise should be like dancing. You're expressing the way you feel. You're reinforcing the feeling of body awareness by sensory feedback from your muscles. You should get good rhythms going, rather than doing militaristic by-the-numbers movements.

Military exercise has two purposes. One is physical training. The other is physiological conditioning. Just as the dress is uniform, so must the movements be uniform. All soldiers move alike, whether or not the same movement is exhausting for some and very light for others. When all do the same movement the same way, the weak are either broken down or conditioned up, and the strong are deconditioned. Eventually all are in the same mediocre condition.

Most exercise routines still reflect the militaristic origins of calisthenics. So do gymnastics, which originated in Germany among farm workers seeking fitness for war. They designed routines using farm implements. Gymnastics today are Teutonic; the competitor is taught to be erect and rigid, like a soldier, and come to a precise position when he dismounts.

If someone asks you to do an exercise, you immediately feel that you must do it properly, which means rigidly and formally. This is just one more example of a misguided emphasis on the physical part of exercise, what you are doing, rather than on its internal effect, what's being done to you. It's the internal effect you're after. If you're a competitive gymnast, then you have to perform formally to get points. But if you're exercising in your bedroom, what you want to do is stretch and get your heart rate going, put a little load on your muscles and get them into tone. No one's giving *you* points for the way you look, or the number of times you do something. We're not looking at the stopwatch. It's not the beat of your clock but the beat of your heart that's important.

DO YOUR OWN THING

Fitness exercise has only one purpose: physiological conditioning—to improve and maintain body functions such as muscular strength and endurance, and circulo-respiratory endurance. Parade-ground uniformity is not necessary: there is no set rhythm, distance, time, position, or range of motion. The individual adjusts each parameter to his own requirements. He moves as he feels like it, according to his own ideas.

Now, this is not to say that group harmony in movement is bad; close-order drill, like singing or dancing in a well-directed chorus, can be a transcending experience for those who enjoy it. But its main purpose is not personal development. In fitness exercises one marches to the beat of one's own drum.

The toughest jobs I have are to convince people, first, that they shouldn't try to lose more than one pound a week—we'll go into that subject extensively in Chapter V—and, second, that they should exercise according to their own inner rhythm. At the outset of World War II, I went to Terminal Island in San Francisco to take a course for prospective naval commanding officers. My background in physical education was duly noted, and I was asked to lead the exercises. We had been doing ordinary calisthenics: toe touching, jumping jacks, and so forth. The first thing I did was tell everyone to sit down. Then I explained to them that since they were going to be aboard ship in confined quarters, they would need an exercise routine they could do in their cabins. I outlined these cabin exercises, and then I asked each man to try them, working out according to his own rhythm and stopping when he felt like it. The officer was horrified. If one of his superiors should come along and see the men doing exercises in such a sloppy way, there would be hell to pay. So we went back to the military, by-the-numbers routines. They looked very good to the observer, but they didn't give much benefit to the practitioner.

Recently I came in contact with one of my fellow officers, Steve Miller, now a stockbroker. He told me that he was still doing his cabin exercises, but hadn't done any calisthenics since he left the Navy thirty years ago.

During the war, naval air cadets were put through the most severe fitness program imaginable and carried to an extremely high level of fitness. But a year after they were on duty, they had reverted to their old sedentary paunchiness. The only exercise they took was elbow bending at the officers' club. They'd been soured on fitness. Military training programs haven't been the same since.

Fliers are individualistic. They resist regimentation. They're the most outspoken against physical training. They see the need to be fit. But they, like me, hate exercise of a regimented type. In 1948, I went to the Air Force School of Aviation and Research in San Antonio to establish a program that would relate physical fitness to flying performance. I will never forget the protest of one major: "For Christ's sake, Dr. Morehouse, you don't have to be able to lift the plane in order to fly it." I agreed.

When the astronaut program was being developed, there were several attempts by Air Force doctors and physical-fitness experts to devise a rigid physical-training program for the spacemen. The first astronauts were test pilots, the most independent of all fliers. They flatly refused to be regimented. Their argument was that each could exercise on his own and prepare himself in his own way for the expected rigors of space flight. It was an excellent argument—and it applies no less to you.

The surest way to get your exercise accomplished is to do it on your own. You won't waste time getting to and from a gym. You won't have to strip and shower an extra time each day. You can fit your workout into your daily pattern.

The one thing that should be firm in your mind before you start is what you hope to accomplish. I learned a great lesson in this regard from John Smith, a UCLA runner who held the world's record in the quarter mile. Every time he goes out for a workout, he has an objective in mind. It may be just one thing, but it's specific. Until he began to work out in this manner, he was getting nowhere; once he adopted the practice, he rose to world class. Your objective should be to make a little more intensive effort than you did the previous session, to be able to maintain that level of exertion for an extra few seconds, or raise your heartbeat an extra few strokes a minute, or develop a certain segment of your body.

Above all, you should choose the things that you enjoy doing, rather than those you must compel yourself to do. You should never feel that you are forcing yourself to exercise.

Exercise can be defined as a specific set of movements to achieve a specific goal. If you do those movements by doing a fast tango, you've gotten the bulk of your exercise. There are certain requirements that have to be met. If you don't meet them, you won't be fit. But you could meet them every day without ever doing one solitary exercise.

IV

What Happens When You Do
—and If You Don't

You may have heard the story of the *nouveau riche* lady who drives up to a resort hotel in a big new convertible. "You carry the suitcases," she tells one of the bellhops. "You carry the trunk," she tells a second. "And you," she tells a third, "carry my son."

The third bellhop regards the twelve-year-old boy. "What's the matter, lady, can't he walk?" he demands.

"Yes, he can walk," she responds, "but, thank God, he doesn't have to."

The truth, of course, is that the person who ceases to walk soon loses his ability to do so.

If man is provided with a favorable environment, an abundance of food, a nice ambient climate and easy sex, his level of fitness will diminish to the level needed for survival. But let that ambience change, and he becomes disturbed and fearful. "I exist only as I am capable of meeting demands of my environment," he tells himself. "If I'm dependent, I'm in a dangerous state."

Fitness is nothing more nor less than adaptation

to the environment. Because man has intelligence, he can determine the degree of his adaptation. He is fit for the sedentary life that characterizes most of his activities, but he has the intelligence to say, "I want to be fit enough to have some fun with my body." He also realizes that he can't stay as weak as the sedentary life makes him, and get away with it forever. There comes a time when he has to do some fighting, climbing or straining for which he won't be fit if he doesn't train.

We once thought that physical activity added to the wear and tear on the body tissues and advanced the aging process. We know now that the opposite is true. Body tissues and functions are improved by physical activity. Continued use delays the aging process. Use makes the organ—the heart, the bones, even the sexual organ.

Body structures and functions adjust to the load placed on them. When the load is diminished, muscles waste away and strength is lost. The heart becomes smaller, weaker and less efficient. Blood vessels disappear. Less is stored of energy chemicals. As a result, the body becomes less capable of meeting physical demands, and may fail in emergency situations. Mild heart attacks, strokes and metabolic disorders such as diabetes are more likely to have devastating consequences.

Perhaps the best proof yet of the effects of inactivity has come from the experiences of our astronauts. Those who took the first week-long trips in space lost ten percent of their bone. During the fourteen-day trip, bone deterioration rose to fifteen percent. We began to wonder whether men could go to the stars, after all. Would there be anything left of them when they got there? But in the Skylab missions, we discovered that after fifty days, deterioration began to level off. The astronauts reached a plateau of fitness that was lower than the one they started with, but definitely adequate to accomplish their jobs in space. In the Apollo missions we learned that the astronaut who remained in lunar orbit in the command capsule deteriorated more than the astronauts who went onto the moon's surface and worked.

WHY EXERCISE HELPS THE HEART

Most people appreciate that exercise is good for the heart, if only because they've heard the idea propounded so often in recent years. What they may not appreciate—because they haven't been told —is *why* exercise is good for the heart.

With proper exercise, the heart becomes richer in oxygen, more massive and powerful, and more efficient. The reconditioned heart beats more slowly at rest and during work, and acquires a greater pumping capacity.

During relaxation, the heart swells with blood. When the heart pumps, it must push against the load to force the blood out. This is the best exercise the heart can get.

If you want to demonstrate the action of the heart muscle as it wrings the blood out, place the fingers of your left hand in the palm of your right hand.

Now squeeze those fingers with your right hand. The muscles of the heart—represented by the fingers of the right hand—must push against the blood supply—represented by the fingers of your left hand —to force it out of the heart and into the veins. The more blood there, the more the heart must push and the better workout it gets.

The difference between a heart that has been strengthened by this workout and another that hasn't been can be demonstrated in the same manner. Once more, place the fingers of one hand in the palm of the other. Now squeeze the fingers gently. Next, squeeze them hard. The gentle squeeze is precisely the action of a weak heart squeezing blood out of its chamber and into your system. The hard squeeze is a strong heart at work. The difference should be apparent: the heart made strong by exercise will pump blood more efficiently and with less strain.

There's yet another dividend. Exercise provides the heart with a fantastic support system. Every muscle is an auxiliary heart, helping to pump blood. When a muscle contracts, it squeezes blood toward the heart. When it relaxes, it allows the muscle to be filled with blood—exactly like the heart. The muscular man who is fifteen pounds over his normal weight because his muscles are so heavy is not straining his heart with those extra pounds; they are actually working in support of the heart. The man who is fifteen pounds overweight because he's fat is taxing the heart; not only is his flab doing nothing to assist the flow of blood, it possesses millions of parasitic capillaries that need to be serviced with blood by the heart.

A few years ago, I participated in a panel about exercise and the heart with the late Paul Dudley White, the cardiologist who had treated President Eisenhower. We were discussing the relationship between skeletal muscle and heart muscle, when Dr. White said, "Larry, before I consider heart surgery, I always feel the patient's thigh. If the thigh is firm, I know the surgeon is going to find a strong heart to work on when he gets inside. But if the thigh is flabby, the heart's going to be the same—and he's going to have problems."

The proper conditioning exercise is a rhythmic continuous one in which the muscles pump repetitively. As blood pumps from the muscles, it is always toward the heart. We call this action "venous return." Muscle involvement increases the action. A fast heartbeat by itself, without muscle involvement, doesn't do the job. The heart beats rapidly when you're emotional, but you don't get benefit from it because your muscles aren't pumping a larger volume of blood toward your heart, as they do when you exercise. As a consequence, the heart is unloaded; it has no extra blood supply to squeeze against. A fitness workout loads and expands the heart with additional blood, and prepares it for a strong contraction.

The heart is not made to work by itself. You can prove this with a simple experiment. Just stand quietly without moving a muscle. Within a few minutes—five at most—you'll begin to feel faint. Wiggle your toes at once. (If you don't, you'll fall to the floor.) That slight action will contract the muscles of your lower legs and move your blood supply back to your heart from your lower extremities, where gravity has concentrated it. What this experiment proves is that without the support of the skeletal muscles, the heart will not adequately maintain circulation. If you're standing still, the brain will be deprived of blood, and you'll faint.

To the extent that you're not exercising, you're duplicating this experiment. You're relying on the heart to do an amount of work for which it was not designed. It just doesn't have the capacity. The most striking aspect of the experiment is the minute amount of exercise needed to maintain normal circulation. A mere wiggling of the toes corrects the imbalance. It's the same in normal life. The merest amount of physical activity puts the skeletal muscles and the heart muscle in concert. The skeletal muscles become what they were intended to be —auxiliary hearts.

There's an auxiliary lesson here, too. It's a good idea to move around every so often when you're working at a desk or reading in a chair. Your work will be keener for it. I've found that my doctoral students taking four-hour examinations perform in direct proportion to the amount of moving around they do. Those who sit in an all-but-dormant manner throughout the exam start out strong, but invariably the quality of their answers to later questions is below that of earlier answers. Those students who fidget a great deal during the exams, by contrast, respond at a uniform level throughout. The difference is that the fidgeters are getting a more adequate supply of blood to their brains. Those of you familiar with the Quiz Kids will remember how they used to squirm. How distressing that teachers chastise squirmers and extol the immobile students.

Muscles are the engines that move you. The fuels for the engines are chemicals the body constantly renews. These fuels are useless unless they have engines that are capable of functioning. If you don't use a muscle, it wastes away until it all but disappears. Each fiber shrinks to almost nothing. Yet the moment you start to use it again, it's like breathing on a bed of coals. It lights up, ignites. If you're one who has let himself go for twenty years, just try walking around the block. It's like a miracle. Where you thought there was nothing, strength reappears.

If you were to exercise in a laboratory, you would soon see the effects of endurance exercise recorded on instruments—improved physical efficiency, lessened cardiac stress, lessened angina pectoris, more activity without pain, reduced total peripheral resistance in blood circulation, lowered systolic and diastolic blood pressure, increased lumen of arteries increased number of capillaries and lower blood lipids, especially triglycerides. Had you been a cardiac patient, exercise would soon enable you to resume normal activity.

WHY CARDIOLOGISTS EXERCISE

When you don't use blood vessels, they close up, shrink and all but disappear. The moment you re-commence activity, they gradually re-form into vessels, enlarge and reassume their function. One of the reasons that cardiologists are now recommending exercises for the prevention of heart disease and for return to normal activity after a heart attack is the increase in capillarization that exercise produces. Cardiologists theorize that a well-conditioned heart will have more capillaries to take over if and when there's a stoppage of a blood vessel.

In many ways, the symptoms of chronic heart failure are similar to those that accompany heavy exercise. The heart beats faster, the ventilation of the lungs is increased, and the blood can't supply enough oxygen to the tissues. Training for exercise which accustoms the body to rapid heart rate, high lung ventilation and large volumes of oxygen consumption may help the body to cope with a heart attack, should one occur.

There may be no clinical proof as yet that exercise prolongs life, but there is no evidence whatever that it hurts it, and there's an immense amount of suggestive material to indicate that it probably enhances your chances of living longer.

Surgeons and cardiologists treating people with terminal diseases recognize that those who are physically fit at the onset of illness are able to maintain a normal life style in the face of disease for a much longer time than those who aren't fit. And they survive surgery better.

Every cardiologist I know is exercising.

Dr. James Jackson, a surgeon, keeps his diabetes under control with a well-balanced program of insulin injections, sugar intake and exercise. At home he pedals his stationary bicycle exerciser at a heart rate of 140 for twenty continuous minutes every day—a hard workout which he happens to enjoy. On good days he jogs outdoors, monitoring his heart rate to adjust his "dose" of exercise. Not long ago he was planning a trip around the world to address several medical conventions. He was going to be away for over a month, staying in hotel rooms. He would have liked to take his bicycle with him, but of course he couldn't, so he asked me to give him a program. Again I dug out my "cabin exercises" and adjusted them to his regimen. He didn't mind running in place, so after his warmup and muscle-toning exercises he checked his pulse every two minutes while he ran in place for his usual time. By keeping up his exercise this way he didn't have to change his insulin dosage or adjust his diet. And he kept himself in his regular state of excellent physical condition. He now prescribes a similar program for his patients during their rehabilitation from surgery.

Some physicians who are themselves marathon runners believe that such long runs actually give immunity against coronary heart disease.

Medical studies of the risk factors in heart disease do not weigh the lack-of-exercise factor as heavily as they do high blood pressure, cigarette smoking, and high blood cholesterol, but the studies always include exercise in their recommendations of life-style elements that reduce the risk of heart disease.

When a sedentary person becomes fairly active by adding a mild exercise such as walking, many changes take place in his body that can be inferred to be important in developing his resistance to cardiovascular disease. Blood pressure is lowered, resting heart rate decreases, muscles—including the heart muscle—become stronger, there is a vast increase in the number of active small blood vessels which carry blood to the cells of the muscular tissues. The blood itself is improved; it carries more oxygen, and the blood platelets, which become sticky and plug up vessels in the heart and brain, thereby causing heart attacks and strokes, become less sticky with exercise training.

EXERCISE AND LONGEVITY

If active people have all of these advantages, they should have fewer heart attacks—and should live longer, right? Well, they should, and probably do, but epidemiological studies of large populations have not yet clearly differentiated the life spans of active and inactive people. When they do, active people should pay less for life insurance.

The reason why the relation between exercise and longevity will probably never be clear is that the level of activity needed to protect against killer disease is so low that it is almost impossible to define a control group. Almost everyone becomes somewhat active once in a while. And active people become sedentary now and then. This problem of the investigators is no problem to us in planning better life styles, however. We know enough right now not to wait until the epidemiologists get their studies in order. The facts we need are in; if we don't exercise regularly we are hurting ourselves, lessening our capacity for living, reducing the number of active years in our lives, and probably shortening our life span.

We have yet another thing to learn from medical investigations of exercise and heart disease. Recently there were a series of attempts to do fairly long-term studies of the effectiveness of aggressive exercise in lowering the incidence of coronary heart disease. These investigators set the scale of exercise so high and made the regimens so severe that only the most hardy of the participants could adhere to it. The investigators lost their subjects long before the studies were completed. What we can conclude has great pertinence for us in establishing a beneficial load of activity: there is no use in forcing yourself into an exercise (or diet) routine you can't stand. I wouldn't be surprised if the failures to comply with such rigid standards did more harm than good to the participants. It is always depressing and irritating to try to keep a commitment you know you are not going to be able to honor. When you finally drop out you feel guilty and inadequate. These are not good feelings; they are the kind that give you ulcers—and high blood pressure.

The answer: set your standards low enough so that you can live comfortably. Better to be content with taking a little walk every day than to join a jogging group you know you don't belong in. That's why I advocate an exercise program that isn't too tough to take. Your heart must be in it.

THE QUALITY OF LIFE

The process of living has two dimensions. One is the sheer number of days of life. The other is the *quality* of life. There is no doubt that you'll live your days better if you exercise.

Shortly after World War II, when I was at the fatigue laboratory of the Graduate School of Business Administration at Harvard, an executive of a leading corporation approached my study group with a special request. "I feel that those of us who represent management and stockholders are losing out in our bargaining with labor on the basis of sheer physical force," he said. "Our bargaining sessions are marathon affairs. Management's representatives invariably smoke and drink too much, don't get enough exercise and don't sleep well. On the other side of the table are the blue-collar guys. They've done manual labor. They're physically tough. Let's say we've been meeting since eight in the morning, and now it's ten at night, and we're nearing some compromises. Both sides know it, but our side is dragging. Our lungs are burning. We feel unraveled. Here are these guys on the other side, vigorously pounding the table. I have a feeling that their physical force is overpowering us. Invariably, that's the moment when they make their point, we weaken and they come out with a better contract." The executive held up his hands in resignation. "Is there something we can do to get ourselves physically in shape so we can do our jobs better?"

When someone approaches a scientist with a problem like that, he rarely gets away. We set up a physical-fitness program for men of executive age, and enlisted some corporate officers from Boston as well as some Harvard professors. We tested them on a treadmill to make certain they were receiving a conditioning effect from their efforts. To a man, they showed improvement. The executive who had come to us originally not only showed changes in his lab tests, but also noted a change in his late-afternoon performance on the job. As he explained it, "Before you got me into shape I was operating on the top half of my low capacity, and often worked to my extreme limit. That really dragged me down. Now, with my reserves increased, I can do the same work within the lower half of my capacity. I can produce twice as much without ever approaching my limit. If I get a little tired, a spot of rest will pick me up. I no longer have a tough time getting out of bed mornings. Most important, my increased reserve gives me greater confidence in everything I do. I'm never going to be half a man again." I don't know if he had better luck at the bargaining table, but I'm sure that he would.

FITNESS AND SEX

One of the immediate effects of fitness is what it does to one's performance in bed, first as to frequency and second as to quality. The more responsive your organism, the more heightened your sensual sensations. If you're fatigued and flabby, your response will match your physical state. But it's more than your sensory apparatus. Sex is a strength and endurance event. It makes demands on the neuromuscular and cardiovascular systems. There is a certain muscular fatigue from sexual postures. Perhaps the most demanding aspect of sex from a physiological point of view is that it produces an elevated heart rate and blood pressure. If you're out of shape, your performance will suffer.

When I was at the University of Iowa, I inaugurated a faculty conditioning program. One day, the wife of a professor of Spanish came to me and told me the following story. "Alberto has been under terrific tension. After his teaching, committee work and research, he comes home every night and tries to work on a book. Invariably, he's too tired. He dozes at his desk. But he's so overwrought that when he comes to bed, he can't fall asleep. We've had good sex during the first years of our marriage, but now it's good only on holidays. I feel deprived. Can you help?" I suggested that Alberto call me. The next day he did.

He said he needed to relax, so I enrolled him

in my faculty conditioning program. Each professor was given specific exercises for his deficiencies, in addition to warmup calisthenics and a swimming program that extended him just a tiny bit each session. Alberto received nothing specific for his sexual deficiencies—nor, as it turned out, did he need anything. As the professor's wife confided to me weeks later: "Wow!"

What Alberto received, in addition to extra energy, was a new concept of his masculinity. Forgotten muscles filled out and became firm. He was again proud of what he saw in the mirror.

When a person has been put out of physical activity because of a heart attack or some other disabling disease, he never feels that he's whole again until he can resume sexual activity. It doesn't matter what else he can do; if he can't do that, he's not recovered. Once he can, he is.

Even among healthy people, there is no greater measure of manness or womanness than one's ability in bed. A person who is healthy—free of illness—may nonetheless be unfit for satisfactory sexual relations. The contrary is beautifully true. Herbert De Vries, a USC exercise physiologist and a former student of mine, did a series of studies on residents of Leisure World in Southern California. He found that exercise lessened the depressive states often found in older people—and that those with higher fitness scores also reported a more satisfactory sexual life in their later years.

If you like yourself as a physical being, this enables you to relate more readily to others. You're more willing to have them look at you, touch you and have relations with you. If you don't feel good about yourself, you can't send effective signals to another person. Those signals are sex appeal.

If you only do some exercise, then, you'll get something more out of life. You'll look somewhat younger, feel somewhat better and probably live longer than you would have had you done no exercise at all. If you don't exercise, you're taking the risk of becoming a dependent organism. When a demand is made on you, you'll have to depend on someone else to do your job. If no one does, you won't survive.

Given the alternatives, the choice seems easy. If your psychological perspectives are in order, you'll want to get fit. Nature has made a provision for that by giving the organism fantastic adaptability, so that you can upgrade your condition in a few days to a point where you will no longer be prostrate in the face of demands.

If looking and feeling better, and probably living longer, aren't sufficient arguments, there is yet another to consider. Exercise is the key to painless and permanent loss of flab—the excess fat we accumulate when we slacken.

V

How To Lose Weight Forever Without Torturing Yourself in the Process

Weight control is the most abused problem in the field of personal maintenance. Millions of pudgy innocents, captives of standards that have no relationship to reality, are seduced by a few dozen charlatans—doctors, physical therapists and nutritionists, among them—with promises that can't be kept. Popular fad diets and crash programs are, for the most part, torturous, dangerous and worthless.

Yet weight control is just as easy to achieve as is muscular and cardiovascular endurance. I said at the outset that you don't need to starve yourself or eliminate foods of any kind. I'll say now that if you do either you're defeating your objective.

If you decide to make the pulse-count fitness guide an integral part of your life, then weight control will be as simple as saying no to an extra piece of toast in the morning and an extra ounce of Scotch at night.

I've helped a thousand people lose weight. As I indicated earlier, the hardest part has been to con-

vince them that they should not—indeed, *must not*
—lose more than a pound a week. That's fifty-two
pounds a year, enough, surely, to satisfy anyone.
Despite my admonitions, many of them have decided to go faster. Every one who has has failed.
Those who adhere to the program invariably suc-
ceed. They are bound to. The process is automatic.
There is no possibility of failure. *If* you are a bit
more active and *if* you make a tiny adjustment in
your caloric intake, you've got to lose weight. There
is no other way to lose weight permanently without injuring your body.

The system is so absolutely certain, in fact, that
it requires you to *gain* weight if you get ahead of
schedule. Only a scheduled weight loss will endure.

Now let me prove these statements.

The human body works exactly like an engine.
It obeys the laws of physics, principally the law of
conservation of energy. The energy that translates
into work must first enter the body as food. When
a person uses more energy than he receives in
caloric food content, he *must* lose weight. It's a
physical principle. So is the opposite case. When
a person takes in more caloric food content than he
expends in energy, he *must* gain weight. The av-
erage-sized adult eats about 2,400 calories a day.
He uses about 2,300 calories a day. This 100-
calories-a-day difference between intake and use
is the cause of his creeping obesity.

HOW TO HALT CREEPING OBESITY

Let's suppose you're this average person. Look at how close you are to altering the balance in your favor. With just a 100-calorie adjustment, you can halt creeping obesity. You can make the adjustment in two ways—either by eliminating 100 calories (one cup of coffee with cream and sugar, or one ounce of cheese) or by burning an extra 100 calories of energy (fourteen minutes of tennis, twenty minutes of gardening).

Once you're even, one more adjustment of either kind will mean that you're using more calories than you're ingesting. At that moment, your body—which must still run on fuel—begins to use its stores of energy. Suddenly, you're burning fat.

Fat cells in the body are the storage bins of excess food intake. Their purpose is for emergencies. In primitive times, when hunters couldn't find game for a week, they could fall back on their fat cells to provide them with the energy they needed to keep hunting. Today, with food readily available, fat storage is unnecessary. The only advantage to carrying extra fat is if you intend to make a long-distance cold-water swim across the English Channel, or if you play a contact sport and want the fat to cushion severe blows to your body. The disadvantages are crippling. The fat person is encumbered, unattractive and vulnerable.

Fat is rich in blood vessels. With every extra pound of fat, miles of new blood vessels are laid down. To receive a blood supply, these vessels have to draw blood away from other body organs. This demand places a strain on the heart. That's why the overweight person doesn't have the life expectancy he would have if he were lean.

If the penalties are so severe, why do intelligent people, presumably eager to live as long a life as they can, permit themselves to become fat?

It's not entirely their fault.

A newborn baby has all the right reflexes. When he's hungry, he cries for his mother. He gets fed. When he's satisfied, he stops feeding. He won't take any more. You can stuff the nipple into his mouth, and he may hold it, but he won't suck. He thrives. His inner mechanism directs him perfectly in his struggle for survival.

Then something happens to upset the balance. Sometimes there is nothing more dangerous and unhealthful than a loving mother. Father, nurse and teacher are willing accomplices. Between them, they literally pollute the baby. They reward him for overeating. They praise his bowel movements. They destroy his natural program.

We are all polluted babies. We continue to reward ourselves as adults in the same way we were rewarded as babies. "Finish your plate" becomes "You must have some more." Never mind that we're not hungry, or already overweight; if someone has cooked something for us, we feel obligated to eat it. Or, because lunchtime has certain well-established rituals, we adhere to them even though we may not need it, or want to. Thanksgiving celebrates the absence of starvation; we're expected to eat until we burst.

The first step in any program of weight therapy is to recognize that we are as we are because of a conditioning process impressed upon us by well-meaning parents, friends and teachers. Because we were taught to eat a certain way doesn't mean we must continue.

But recognition alone can't solve problems. We must understand their components as well.

WHAT SCALES DON'T TELL YOU

When you weigh yourself, you must be able to interpret what you read.

It's not fat you're measuring when you step on the scale. You can actually lose weight and gain fat. That happens frequently to athletes at the end of a season of competition. They cease to work hard, yet keep eating the same amount. Their muscles atrophy. Because muscle weighs much more than fat, the loss in muscles shows up as a loss of weight on the scale. So the athletes are actually losing weight while gaining fat. But their scales don't tell them that.

Nor do scales indicate the extent of residues in the body that are going to be eliminated within a short period. Let's suppose you've eaten four pounds of food in one meal. This may register as three pounds the next morning. That's a horrifying sight when seen on the scale, but it's a misreading of your condition. Three days later, the excess food and water will have been all but excreted. Your real weight gain from that fiesta will be no more than a pound—if that. And if you've eaten conservatively in the interval and been fairly active, you'll be right back where you were before you indulged.

Scales don't interpret weight gain attributable to climate. On humid days, the body absorbs moisture to such a degree that scale weight increases as much as one and a half pounds. Playing golf in desert air can cause a scale weight loss of three to five pounds in one day. Neither the gain nor the loss is permanent.

A bathroom scale is not a precision instrument. The pointer doesn't return to zero each time after you've weighed, or to the same reading when you step back on again. The kind of engineering that degree of accuracy requires would make scales too expensive for home uses. Even when your dial registers zero, your weight won't necessarily be measured in the same way it was the day before. Just by shifting your weight around, or standing in a different position, you can cause the dial to move as much as five pounds in one direction or the other. By accepting your bathroom scale as your master, you indenture yourself to a vacillating tyrant.

If you weigh yourself daily, and you're steadily gaining weight, it could mean an increase in muscle weight caused by heavy work or exercise. If you haven't done any muscle building, then you can assume the weight gain is fat. If you're losing weight, on the other hand, the scale can't assure you that what you're losing is fat. The weight loss may be caused by dehydration, excessive urination due to an intake of diuretic fluids like tea or beer. Weight-reduction programs that promise losses of five pounds a week and more are usually based on scale weight, and rely on diuresis. This can't be considered weight loss in terms of fatty weight. The scale weight will return to its former reading almost as soon as you begin to replace the fluid.

If it were possible to eat exactly the same food every day for ten days, and to have exactly the same amount of physical activity every day, and to be in the same mood and state of tone (between tension and relaxation) and in the same atmosphere (temperature and humidity) you would still have a variation in body weight from day to day. This would be due to the digestive and metabolic processes, which have their own rhythm. You wouldn't defecate the same amount every morning, or urinate the same amount, or lose the same amount of insensible perspiration.

Scales are useful only in giving you a general idea as to your overnutrition. A far better "scale" is your appearance in a mirror. You don't need a weight scale to tell you when you're fat. You can see the pendulous masses hanging on your body, or the flesh jiggle when you move. If folds of fat hang over your belt, you need no further confirmation of your problem. Participants in one faculty conditioning program call this Dunlaps Disease—"Your belly dun laps over your belt."

A NEW STANDARD: OVERWAIST FOR MEN; AN INCH OF PINCH FOR WOMEN

Obesity is a problem of fat, not weight. The generalization that being overweight is the same as being fat, can be misleading. Bulky muscles can add to weight, but people with those muscles may have very little fat on their bodies. We need an added standard to help us gauge our condition.

The object of weight reduction is to lose excess fat without reducing your lean tissues: your muscles, bones and blood. All of these tissues increase with exercise training. While you're losing fat you're gaining valuable tissue. On the scales, your weight may go up instead of down, because the useful tissue you're gaining weighs more than the fat you're replacing. But take a look in the mirror!

It's the fat in your waistline, hips and thighs you should look at, not the poundage on your scale. The true index is your belt size and your skirt or pants size. As fat comes off, these sizes diminish. When your skirt or pants get tight, you're getting fat. When they become loose, you're losing fat. You can forget the scales if you wish, and look solely at your waist. The body weight can be solid muscle. If it's not, your waistline will tell you.

For men particularly, the question is not whether they're overweight, it's whether they're *overwaist*. Men characteristically distribute their fat around their center of gravity when they start to put on weight.

Measuring the waist with a tape measure can give

a highly inaccurate reading unless certain practices are followed. The abdomen must be in a normal state, neither sucked in nor pushed out. The pelvis must be level. The tape must be placed at the belt line, just above the crests of the pelvis, and be horizontal all around. The best method is not to put the tape around your waist, but to use a belt; take in the notches of the belt until it fits snugly but not tightly, then remove the belt and measure it.

But in the case of men a tape measure isn't really necessary. There's a simpler measure yet—the size underwear that they buy. If you are a man who weighs 170 and you can't comfortably get into a size thirty-five brief, then you're carrying too much fat. You needn't be more specific than that.

Fatness Guideline (Men)

If your nude weight is	Your waistline girth should not exceed
(pounds)	(inches)
100	30
110	31
120	32
130	32
140	33
150	34
160	34 *okay*
170	35 *okay*
180	36 *not okay*
190	36
200	37
210	38
220	38
230	39
240	40
250	40

For men, we can actually make up a table comparing their weight to their waistline girth. To find out how you measure up, simply draw a line between weight and waist size. If the line slopes down, you're fat. A level line, or one sloping up, means your waist is okay.

Men have a fairly uniform body construction, and a fairly uniform distribution of fat throughout their bodies. As a consequence, when two men whose normal weight should be the same suddenly begin to gain weight, one because he's gaining fat, the other because he's gaining muscle, the first will gain in the waist, and the second won't.

Women are another matter. Their contours differ widely. They have no regularity of fat distribution. It can accumulate around their thighs or buttocks or breasts or arms. Women who become fat in their lower bodies can remain fairly thin on top.

For women, the best measure of fat is the *inch of pinch* test.

An inch of pinch means about forty pounds of fat in most adults. That doesn't mean you have forty pounds of excess fat; it simply means that of your total weight, forty pounds is fat. Each extra quarter inch in a double fold of skin equals ten pounds of extra fat. Here's how you measure:

Find a book that's exactly one inch thick, measured by a ruler. Get acquainted with the feel of the book between your thumb and your index finger. Then grab the flesh at the side of the belly, the waist, the thigh, the buttocks, the back of the arm. At no point on the body should the skin-fold thickness exceed one inch. If it's more than that, we've got work to do.

THE PERILS OF STARVATION

Not long ago, the wife of a friend of mine decided to lose fifteen pounds. It had taken her a long time to work up her resolve. She determined to get it over with as quickly as she could. She had some energy pills her doctor had prescribed for a previous effort. She took these and very little else.

The first day her scales registered a four-pound loss, the next day another two. Each day thereafter she showed a loss anywhere from half a pound to two pounds. In ten days, she was within three pounds of her goal—at which point she went out to play tennis with her husband. Half an hour after they began, she had to quit. On the way home, her face grew dark red. She began to sneeze and suffer progressive flu-like symptoms. It was a classic reaction to combined starvation and dehydration.

Fasting is a convenient way to lose weight if your body can tolerate it. Some persons can go on a water-only diet for a day or two without detriment. Others with more sensitive carbohydrate metabolic systems have great difficulty if they go more than twelve hours without food.

The objective of any program that combines activity with a restriction of food is to use the body's fat as food. The fat cells provide energy for activity; they're consumed in the process. So long as you're on a very slight deficit regimen and eating a balanced diet, you won't have any problems. But cut out any ingredients, and you're in trouble. Cut out carbohydrates, for example, and you begin to use your body tissues for fuel—not simply fat but muscle and blood stores as well. If you keep at it for long enough, as my friend's wife did, then your carbohydrate is used up and you begin to operate on fat and protein. This produces an acid condition, which is not only an abnormal state, but makes you feel uncomfortable and ill.

Proteins are the building blocks of the body. Both fat and carbohydrate are expendable, but protein is not. Any dietary regimen that forces you to summon protein as a major source of energy is destroying the basic fiber of your existence. Long-term low-carbohydrate diets force the body to use protein for fuel.

The body is always using carbohydrate, protein and fat in its metabolism. Metabolism is composed of two parts—catabolism and anabolism. Catabolism is the breaking down and utilization of substances and tissues in the body. It's a normal process that goes on all the time, and at a normal rate. Anabolism is a continuous building up of the body tissues at a fairly constant rate. If you are in a stable breakdown-buildup cycle, the processes balance each other and your body composition remains uniform. You can increase the catabolic processes by overexertion and starvation, but you can't increase the anabolic processes to the same degree. Instead, your body dips into proteins, even when your diet is high in proteins. Overnutrition and prolonged rest do not markedly accelerate the anabolic processes. They go on at about the same rate.

Our objective is to preserve the body in its normal state. Excess fat has resulted from a little too much rest, not quite enough physical activity, and a little too much food. We want to trim down the food and gear up the activity at the gentle rate that permits normal homeostasis—maintenance of the body's metabolic balance.

There's only one way to do that.

INTRODUCING THE WIDE-VARIETY DIET

Variety is literally the spice of life in matters of nutrition.

It's dangerous to eliminate any type of food from your diet. The danger far outweighs the benefits you might gain from emphasizing one particular type of food. A red warning flag should go up any time you read of a diet that calls for the elimination of any kind of food. You're inviting deficiencies. "Avoid" diets are for patients with allergies or other pathological abnormalities. If you adopt one for yourself it's just like going to a sick person's medicine cabinet and eating his pills.

If your recent blood test shows you're running a high cholesterol count, and you've been eating six eggs a day, it would be prudent for you to reduce your intake of eggs. But eggs and their cholesterol are excellent food; they are not poisonous. It would be unwise to eliminate them entirely. Physical activity and nutrition are closely related. If you are supersedentary you have to be supercautious about your diet. You probably should not eat more than three eggs a week. If you want a few more eggs, just be a little more active.

Special reducing diets, such as grapes only, or pears and cottage cheese only, are severely inadequate and will produce illness if you persist in them a month or more. Poor diets are those that restrict the variety of foods so that you're existing on handfuls of "magic" foodstuffs. Recommendations such as no carbohydrates on the one hand and all carbohydrates, such as grapefruit, on the other hand are leading the users to poor nutrition.

The answer is a wide variety of everything. In a cafeteria, the person whose tray has the best diet on it is the one who chooses the widest variety of foods. This can include cake and ice cream. Obviously, it doesn't mean a wide variety of only that kind of food.

If you love beef, eat beef. Eat whatever you want. If you crave bacon, have it once in a while. It's an excellent idea to treat yourself to something you really want at least once a week. That includes a five-hundred-calorie malt, if you are ravenous for one.

The low-calorie plate found today in most restaurants is based on good nutrition because it offers a number of different kinds of food—a piece of meat, cottage cheese, lettuce and fruit. What makes the plate nutritious is not its quantity or quality, but its variety.

A variety of foods means a mixture of carbohydrates, fats, proteins, vitamins and minerals.

Refined carbohydrates, white sugar and white flour, are probably the least nutritious in terms of the useful food substances they contain. Refined carbohydrates are quickly converted into fat if they are taken in excess of the energy used. Much of the cholesterol deposited in the blood vessels of inactive people is thought to be the result of an overabundance of sugar in the diet, rather than fat, as most people believe.

It's a general misconception that the tissue in the body is the result of the type of nutrients you eat. Athletes used to think that if they ate a lot more meat they would put on a lot more muscle. Many still think that way, and eat that way. Others now know better. Protein can be formed from carbohydrates and fat, fat can be formed from carbohydrates and proteins, and carbohydrates can be formed from protein and fat. One source of our protein is steer beef, which comes from an animal that eats grass. Grass is almost pure carbohydrate. When we eat beef we're eating processed grass. This demonstrates the absurdity of the notion that "you are what you eat." Your body magic makes you more than what you eat.

When I was a research assistant in physiology at the University of Iowa's School of Medicine in 1940, there were only half a dozen known vitamins. There was great concern at the time that we should all get our full quota of vitamins. Today we know that there are more than a dozen vitamins. It's not unlikely that in twenty years' time we'll have found that there are more than two dozen vitamins. What, then, is the point of taking pills in known quantity each day in order to be certain that you'll get your quota of vitamins? That suggests a certain overreliance on mankind's knowledge to date. There is only one way to be certain that you'll get all your vitamins, and that is to eat a wide variety of foods—especially those foods such as milk, eggs, grains and fish that we know to be highly nutritious. The vitamins we don't yet know about are undoubtedly in those and other wholesome foods.

The same can be said for minerals. Every month, it seems, a new mineral is found to have great importance for our nutrition. One month it's zinc. Another month it's chromium. We'll soon have a list that includes nearly every element in the chemical tables. Instead of taking them as we would medicine, the best guarantee of getting them all, and in proper quantities, is via the wide-variety diet.

One evening recently, I went to a dinner party. My host couldn't wait to get me out to the kitchen. He proudly showed me a row of bottles and containers. It was the largest private collection of food, vitamin and mineral supplements I had ever seen. I didn't have the heart to tell him that he was wasting his money. If he lived in a barren region of Asia and subsisted on potatoes during an entire winter, he would profit from all of these food supplements. But there is no area of the United States where a wide-variety diet can't be obtained. There is no need for such anxiety about intake, or for compulsive habits.

The threats one hears of the ill consequences of

not taking this vitamin or that mineral every single day just can't be backed up any more than arguments for rigid exercise programs on a daily basis, or a scheduled amount of sleep. You have the body of a hunter in sparse lands. Your body carries ample reserves of everything you need to go for days, if necessary, without anything. About the only thing that needs to be replaced almost daily is water. As back-up for the days when you might not be able to eat sufficiently or nourishingly, your marvelous internal plant can manufacture what it needs from the stuff that's there. Your body can make carbohydrate from protein or fat, protein from carbohydrate or fat, and fat from carbohydrate or protein. Even if you're starving, a few calories of any kind of food will be made into the things you need most for survival. Over the long stretch of weeks and months, a wide variety of foods will replace the rare pieces you've used up.

HOW TO FOOL THE EATING HABIT

You can become "addicted" to breakfast at 7 A.M., lunch at noon and dinner at 6 P.M. Miss a meal and you suffer from "withdrawal" symptoms. The same is true with exercise and sleep. If you played handball every day, you would feel terrible if you missed a day. I know. I was a handball "addict." If you sleep soundly from 11 P.M. to 7 A.M., you'll be miserable the day after you've stayed up until 1 A.M., or were awakened at 5 A.M. and couldn't get back to sleep. Regular habit demands adherence. Things go well until the rhythm is broken. Then we suffer.

The antidote is to disrupt the rhythm once in a while, voluntarily. You can avoid compulsion about eating if you intrude on your compulsive schedule. Be casual; don't be a slave to the clock.

When I fly from Los Angeles to New York, I am constantly fighting "jet lag." I'm fresh at night, dull in the mornings. This is because I've formed the habit of regular bedtime. Not long ago, I determined to do something about it. One week before a scheduled trip east, I deliberately began to vary my hours of retiring and arising. By the time I arrived in New York, my habit had loosened up to a point where I was able to adjust better. The principle applies to eating.

It's not healthy to take health regimens too seriously. If they become all-possessing, they crowd out pleasant experiences. They spoil the party for you, and you spoil it for others. Life without feasts would be a pretty dull existence. During a feast, why spoil it? Don't be conscious of restrictions.

But anticipate indulgence. It's so much easier to restrain yourself knowing you'll be rewarded a few hours hence than it is to cut back the morning after in penance for your sins.

If you have a date for lunch at a good restaurant and you know there will be special things you'll want to eat, take your breakfast a little earlier, or eat smaller portions. If you're invited to dinner at Mom's, plan to be hungry when you get there.

On normal days, the best favor you can do yourself is to have a good breakfast. It sets you up for a hunger-free day.

The best distribution is a substantial breakfast, a moderate lunch and a light supper. Snacks before bedtime seem to be the ones that manufacture fat. It's the calories, not the hour, that make the difference.

If you're carbohydrate-sensitive, meaning that almost any amount of deprivation bothers you, you're undoubtedly familiar with the critical moments when diets go out the window. You feel starved. You're unhappy and uncomfortable to the point of illness. You know you need food, so the hell with it, you eat. And the food tastes and smells and feels so good that you suddenly want to eat everything in sight—and do. Four, five, six, seven hundred, forget it, a thousand calories. That splurge sets you back five days.

Next time you get that feeling, fight fire with fire. Starved for carbohydrate, eat carbohydrate, but don't use a bucketful when a glassful will douse the flames. A small amount of sweet food, such as a glass of cider or an orange, will pick you up almost immediately. If nothing better is around, eat a piece of candy. One piece is enough. You may feel like eating more, but you don't have to. The frantic feeling will soon pass. You'll not only feel satisfied, you'll feel virtuous as well. You won't have wrecked a thing.

To recapitulate: The best possible diet for everyone, athletes included, is a wide variety of foods in quantities necessary to maintain normal body weight. The body is a machine in which the energy taken in must equal the energy used up to achieve equilibrium. Food is potential energy. If you take in more food than you use up, you store it as fat. If you use more than you're taking in, you'll lose some of that stored fat.

FATTEN UP BEFORE YOU REDUCE

When people come to me with a weight problem, I tell them that my program always starts on the following Monday morning—and they have until then to eat up. Until the program starts, I don't want any dietary restrictions. They can eat everything in sight. I deliberately want that weight to be heavy on Monday morning because the first two weeks of any program are the hardest. During that period, they're adjusting their metabolism. Feeding in advance of the program makes the metabolic adjustment easier.

If you want to have a program that fails, you start in a period of semistarvation and try to go down from there. The worst thing you can do when you decide to lose weight is to starve yourself for a week. The only possible good you're doing yourself is to satisfy your guilt. You've sinned, and now you pay penance. If you're fasting as a form of absolution, okay, but it's no good as a reducing method. Fasts are invariably followed by feasts.

My friend's wife—the one who lost twelve

pounds in ten days and then became ill—had thought that by going without food for a couple of days she would shrink her stomach. That's a false notion. What may shrink is the stomach's habit of receiving food, in which case the stomach produces fewer hunger pains. But the actual size of the stomach doesn't change.

Malnutrition had provoked her reaction to physical activity. She had used her meager reserve of carbohydrate, the main source of fuel, at the outset of her tennis match. She became hypoglycemic. Her blood sugar fell below the level needed to maintain brain function. It also made her susceptible to allergies, and infection. I told her husband to get some food into her. She refused. A few days later, she took sick.

The reason she refused seemed plausible enough. "I've gone to all this trouble to lose weight, and I'll be damned if I'm going to put it back on again," she said. But the truth was that she hadn't lost that much fat. Most of her loss was water. Food contains large amounts of water, fifty percent or more. By drastically curtailing her supply of food and beverages, she had deprived her vital body tissues —muscles and nerve and visceral tissues—of needed fluid. The moment she returned to a sensible diet —and she would have to eventually to cure her illness—she would gain back all but one or two of the pounds she had lost.

Eventually, she resumed eating enough to keep her energy up. She had to. She had been on an in-human, biologically unsound program. She had tampered with her normal body processes. She had asked too much of herself to function in a semi-starved condition.

At this point, I offered her four alternatives:

1. She could continue the crash program and hope she had the superior quality of tissues and functions that would withstand such an insult.

2. She could regain half the weight she had lost, and then continue on a more rational fat-loss program.

3. She could maintain her present low weight and try to consolidate it, hoping she could get away with it. She had lost twelve pounds. She could, conceivably, hold the gain if she remained at that weight for a few months.

4. She could regain all her weight and start over —in which case I would guarantee her that if she did what I asked her to do, she would lose the twelve pounds in twelve weeks. And this time it would be permanent.

I told her that I vastly preferred that she gain back the weight. It was a beautiful starting weight.

Grudgingly, she acceded. She had a splendid time working her way back up to the starting point. Then I put her on the program.

CHOOSE A WEIGHT FOR THE REST OF YOUR LIFE

The size and fit of your clothes is still the best index of determining if you're fat, but it's inadequate as a daily guide to fat reduction. For that you need your bathroom scale—as imperfect as it is.

In our program, we act as if the scale were telling the truth about your body's fat percentages. We know variations take place, but by and large we ignore them. On days when humidity or other factors are giving us high scale readings, we act as if that were a true weight gain, and govern ourselves accordingly. The same for dry days when there's a drop in scale weight; we consider that a fat drop. We pay attention to the scale, particularly since it's such a good source of motivation, but we don't take it too seriously.

If you're up when you thought you should be down because you've been so conscientious, blame it on the weather. But keep being conscientious. The factors that put you up will probably be adjusted the following day. But if you're still up the following day, and the day after that, you've lost your excuse, it's undoubtedly fat buildup and you must adjust accordingly.

There are ways to diminish these variables to a minimum.

When you start your program, adjust your scale to zero, seal the adjustment wheel with a piece of tape and don't touch the wheel again until your program is completed. When you stand on the scales, just stand in a comfortable balance, with your weight evenly distributed on both feet. We have a tendency to adjust the scale to where we want it. So don't look at the scale meter as you step on until your feet are in place. When you look down, that's your weight for the day. Don't try to maneuver it.

The Monday morning she was to visit me, my friend's wife, following my instructions, weighed herself nude before breakfast after defecating and urinating. She weighed in at 142.

"Okay," I began, when she got to my office, "how much do you want to weigh for the rest of your life?"

My question startled her. She seemed at a loss.

"You don't have a program until you have an objective," I said. "And it must be a reasonable, moderate, obtainable objective. Pick a weight that you know you can achieve, one that will make you no thinner than when you were in a comfortable state of leanness. Review your body-weight history. Try to remember when you looked and felt your best, and could easily maintain the weight. Your goal is to be *fairly* lean, not lean."

She had weighed as little as 117 in college, but knew that that weight wasn't realistic. She chose a weight she had maintained comfortably for a number of years: 127 pounds.

Next, we took a piece of graph paper and entered her starting weight, 142, near the upper left-hand corner. We made a dot at that point. Each square on the graph, I explained, equaled half a pound in the left-hand margin. Every second square going down the page, we entered the next lower number: 141, 140, 139, etc.

Along the bottom of the paper, we began with the date that day, and numbered each square as one day across the width. Then we returned to the upper left-hand corner and counted seven squares from left to right, beginning at the initial weight of 142.

At the seventh horizontal square, we dropped down two squares, and made a dot, and at the fourteenth and twenty-first dropped down another two squares at each respective point and made the appropriate dots. Using a ruler we then connected the upper left-hand corner to the third of the dots with a line that ran through the other dots as well.

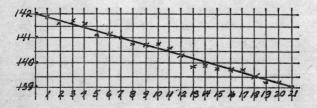

"That's your weight-control program for the first three weeks," I told her. In the first week, and in each week that follows until you reach your desired weight, you lose one pound, no more, no less. So, since you want to lose fifteen pounds, it's going to take fifteen weeks and a total of five three-week charts like this one to carry it out. Since your first chart runs from 142 to 139, the second will run from 139 to 136, the third from 136 to 133, the fourth from 133 to 130, and the fifth from 130 to 127.

"Each day, before breakfast, you weigh yourself nude. That's your weight for the day. You record the weight on the graph paper, either above or below or on the line. *You're not a hero if you're below the line. You're a hero only if you're on the line.*

"If you're below the line, it means that you can

eat as you wish that day in order to raise your weight so that you're on the line the following day. If you're above the line, it means that you're going to have to say no to the food you don't need that day, and that you're going to have to seek a little more physical activity than usual. If that's the day you have a dinner party planned, you can prepare for it by eating half a portion of breakfast and lunch."

"How do you measure fractions of pounds?" she asked.

"Just go to the nearest half pound. It's impossible to control weight to minute amounts. The scales aren't going to be all that accurate. But the weight you record is close enough to serve as the guiding principle of your program."

The key to the success of the program, I explained, was that, unlike her previous experience, she would not have a daily fight. "Some days you're going to be below the line. Go ahead and have that chocolate sundae. Some days you'll be above. On those days, no sundae. You'll be using your body fat as part of your meals, but so little you won't be uncomfortable. This program is rigorous enough for non-Spartan folks like you and me. Anything beyond this becomes a superhuman feat, just more than we can endure. The body will readily adjust to this moderate program, and you'll feel neither starved nor driven. If you attempt to lose a pound a day, you're dedicating yourself to a life of continuous gnawing hunger and depletion of physical vigor. Dieting leads to lethargy in order to conserve energy—just the opposite of what we want to achieve.

The pound-a-week process is one to which you can become habituated."

"What about calories?" she wondered.

"There's no need to count calories. The scales will count them for you. Ignore the possibility that fluctuations in body weight may be due to the weather or unusual activities. Keep trying to bring the weight to the control line every morning, by adjusting food intake and physical activity. After the first week, you'll know almost exactly what the weight cost will be of a dessert or an extra helping.

"Once your proper weight level is reached, continue your morning weighing and adjusting food intake to stay on the control line for at least one week. After that, twice-weekly weight checks before breakfast will monitor the balance between food intake and energy output."

"Okay," she said, "now *how* do I reduce?"

THE POUND-A-WEEK REDUCTION

A pound of fat has 3,500 calories. To lose a pound of fat a day, you would have to use 3,500 calories more than you take in. Unless you eat nothing, and work like a horse, it's impossible. I'm speaking of permanent weight loss in terms of fat, as against temporary weight loss in terms of water.

Even to lose a pound of fat a week, you would need to use five hundred calories a day more than you take in. To exercise this much off every day would be a lot of work. Few of us have the time for it, let alone the inclination.

If, however, you were to combine "caloric burn" from activity together with dietary restraint, you could produce five hundred calories of deficit a day without either strain or starvation—and lose one pound of fat every week.

My formula for permanent weight loss is to diminish daily food intake by two hundred calories and to use three hundred extra calories in physical activity.

With this combination, your metabolism is not upset. All of your body processes are operating in proper chemical balance. Proteins are preserved. Normal "pH"—the range between acidity and alkalinity of the body—is maintained. When you lose a pound with this process you lose not a pound of water or a pound of vital body tissue but a pound of excess fat.

My program can't be compared to programs that promise weight loss of seven pounds in a week. Such programs are successful only if they induce large fluid losses. About sixty percent of the body is water; this amount of water is necessary to maintain normal function of tissues. If you dry out by cutting down your fluid intake, or if you drain out by taking diuretics, or if you sweat yourself out in steam baths or saunas, then you're just putting yourself in a temporary, unnatural state of fluid imbalance. The fluid must quickly be restored or you'll find yourself in poor health.

In these heroic water-loss methods, some fat may be lost, if there is a restriction in caloric intake or an increase in physical activity. Even restlessness or a loss of sleep, which occur when you take stimulants, will bring about some fat loss. But your fatigue will catch up to you in a short time, and you'll be logy for as many days as you were high. When you recover from failure to lose fat after using pills or water-loss methods, you've done well to have come out even.

The caloric cost of exercise for women is roughly the same as for men. Men have heavier bodies and body frames and thus more bulk to move, but women have a higher circulo-respiratory response before, during and after exercise. In general, all adults use about three hundred calories per day more when they increase their activity level from a sedentary to a moderate one.

Like the cruising speed of walking, there seems to be an optimal cruising rate of food intake. Below this intake, you're going to be hungry whether you're active or not. Above it you're going to be obese unless you match the increased intake with increased activity. When you attack the problem piecemeal, it can be tough. It takes an extra mile of walking or running to work off an extra slice of bread and butter.

As physical activity is decreased there is not a concomitant decrease in appetite. In fact, the opposite occurs. Physical inactivity leads to increased food intake. Cattle raisers know this and pen their stock. The result of inactivity is a rapid gain in body fat and a softening of muscle tissue. This makes for tender steaks, but nothing good comes of it for humans. It seems an enviable situation when millions of people are supplied with an over-abundance of food and at the same time have no hard physical work to do. For the majority, the situation is disastrous, because overfeeding and underexercise lead to death-dealing obesity and degenerative disease of the heart and blood vessels.

The key to easy weight loss is to use three hundred activity calories a day above your normal level. If you do that, then your "dieting" really will consist of eliminating nothing more than that extra slice of toast in the morning, or the one extra jigger of Scotch at night. You won't eliminate toast or Scotch or any other food. You'll simply cut down on any two of the many items you consume during the day. Consider the following table.

100-Calorie Food Portions		Minutes of Various Activities to Consume 100 Calories
1 cup coffee with cream and sugar	7	Run 1,500 yards (7.3 mph)
1 griddle cake (pancake)	9	Bicycle 2 miles (13 mph)
¾ cup cream of wheat or flakes	9	Swim 400 yards (45 yards a minute)
2 tablespoons sugar	10	Downhill skiing
1 fried egg	14	Tennis
A 5-ounce glass of milk	20	Golf
¼ cup canned tuna	20	Gardening
1 ounce cheese	20	Walk 1,500 yards (2.6 mph)
½ cup tomato or vegetable soup	22	Bowling

100-Calorie Food Portions		Minutes of Various Activities to Consume 100 Calories
An 8-ounce glass of cola soft drink	31	Washing, showering, shaving, etc.
A ⅔-ounce chocolate bar	80	Reclining in bed
1 ounce Scotch		
2 ounces ground beef		
1 baked potato		
6 potato chips		
5 French-fried potatoes		
1¼ apples		
¹⁄₁₂ quart of ice cream		
2 plain cookies		

It should be immediately evident from a comparison of the two columns that it requires a good deal of isolated exercise to work off one hundred calories. Isolated exercise in sporadic bouts won't work. Joggers often assume that it's just a matter of so many miles, and then they're going to be thin. After forty-five minutes of jogging they've lost two or three pounds, but most of that weight loss is water loss, which will be replaced by a few glasses of water or a few cups of coffee. They assume that because they jogged today, they can have a piece of cake. The piece of cake contains twice the number of calories they burned while jogging.

The jogger may have used only two hundred calories during his workout. If, during the rest of the day, he returns to a sedentary pattern, and he does nothing further about his diet, he'll probably gain weight, not lose. He's done it the hard way, and he's got nothing to show for it.

Most of us aren't runner types. We don't enjoy it. We're not built for it, particularly if we're overweight. Add to this the insult of wearing heavy clothes or impermeable garments to sweat off weight, and we've subjected ourselves to severe punishment. Even the prospect of a reward such as a steady weight loss, assuming it were forthcoming, wouldn't be enough to maintain interest. Adherence to such programs is dismal. Most people drop out after the first week.

There's a better way.

SWAPPING FAT FOR HEALTHY TISSUE

The remainder of this book will be about how to integrate physical activity into your life in such a way that you need do little and possibly nothing at all in the way of special physical exercise in order to use activity calories.

The program is divided into four steps.

In Step One, you'll exchange useless fat for vital muscle, bone and blood, and begin to develop circulo-respiratory endurance.

In Step Two, you'll keep losing fat and expand your muscular and circulo-respiratory endurance.

In Step Three, you'll lose more fat if you need to, and increase your muscular strength and circulo-respiratory endurance.

In Step Four, you'll stabilize your new physical condition: your new level of fat, your lean tissues, your muscular strength and endurance, and your circulo-respiratory endurance.

If you're overweight and underexercised when you start your program, you may not lose weight for a while, because as you build muscle, bone and blood the weight of those vital tissues may disguise the loss of fat. Instead of seeing a noticeable change on your scale, you'll see the loss of fat. You'll be losing weight all the time in your waistline, thighs and hips and the back of your arms. Your clothes will fit less tightly, and your figure will improve. What the scales don't tell you your waistline will. You'll be exchanging flab for lean and solid flesh.

After a couple of months of training, muscle enlargement tapers off. Now the balance between food intake and energy output of physical activity is more accurately revealed by changes in body weight.

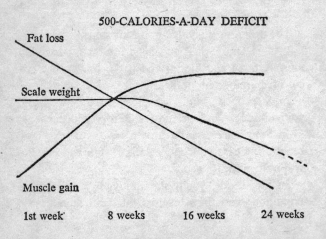

500-CALORIES-A-DAY DEFICIT

Fat loss

Scale weight

Muscle gain

1st week   8 weeks   16 weeks   24 weeks

The weight loss on the scale can now be interpreted as fat loss.

The scales say that you're losing a pound a week. In actuality, you're losing a lot more than a pound of fat. You're gaining weight of a valuable kind—not just muscle, but an increase in your quantity of blood vessels—and you're losing weight of a dangerous kind. Each pound that you lose in this fashion, as measured by your scale, is infinitely more valuable to your health and fitness than the liquid pounds that you might lose in some crash diet.

IV

The Theory of Heart-rated
Exercise

In the mid-1960s, there was a concentrated effort of
the United States Public Health Service, led by
Dr. Samuel Fox, to investigate the role of exercise
in the prevention of America's number-one killer,
coronary heart disease. Dr. Fox brought together a
group of physicians and exercise physiologists; I was
part of that group. I told my colleagues that exercise, in my opinion, had to be approached in an entirely new way before it could effectively condition
the heart. All previous programs had concentrated
on performance. I proposed that we now concentrate on the physiological effect of what people did.
The difference was fundamental. In the old version,
you ran a certain distance in a certain time. In the
new version, you would determine the distance
and the rate you needed to run by the effect it
would produce on your heart. The number of heartbeats per minute could be determined by counting the pulse.

Dr. Fox and the group asked me to perform an
experiment to evaluate the feasibility of my idea to

use pulse rate to monitor exercise. It was the start of the pulse-rated program.

I had been using pulse rate for some time to monitor my own personal fitness program. As a physiologist working in a laboratory where measurements are constantly made, I was accustomed to relying on these measurements to determine how much exercise a person was getting. It occurred to me that the simplest measure of all was the pulse. You just looked at the second hand on your watch and counted the number of pulse beats and you could determine how hard you were exercising. The method worked well for me, but there was some question as to whether it would work equally well among groups. One of my students, Ludmilla Raisters, agreed to find out; she made it her master's-degree project. Ludmilla was then a physical-education teacher in the Torrance, California, high schools. It was my thought that if people as flighty as most high-school girls could be taught to check on the conditioning effect of their workouts, then almost anyone could be taught the same thing.

We didn't know at the outset whether the girls could count their pulse with any accuracy, or what effect the pulse counting would have on their motivation for fitness, or whether they had any interest at all in the cardiovascular effects of exercise. Did they really care whether badminton promoted fitness? Or did they just want to play badminton?

The results were gratifying. Not only were the girls interested in counting their pulse. Not only were their results accurate. They became extremely interested in their cardiovascular systems, the importance of fitness, and how badminton could work as a fitness exercise.

There had been no point in even considering the application of a pulse-rated method until we could learn that people were motivated and could do it. Once we established that, it opened a whole new avenue to fitness. Now we could devise a controlled program to verify the conditioning effect of exercise.

THE TROUBLE WITH PREVIOUS PROGRAMS

In the years before I adopted the pulse-count method, I had increasingly suspected that even I had been exercising improperly. My program incorporated weight training with jogging and cycling. But I had the feeling that how much I lifted or how far I ran wasn't important. Some days the loads I lifted seemed too heavy. Some days they seemed too light. Some days I felt my distance run was too little. Some days it seemed too much.

I began to review all the previous programs by which fitness training was governed. Change in the physiological sciences is a prevalent characteristic. As just one small measure of how swiftly our understanding of fitness keeps changing, my textbook, which is the standard text on the subject of exercise physiology for colleges and universities, has to be revised every three years. By the time I have assembled the revision, I already have new data suggesting that what I've written will need to be revised. So it was very much in order for me to review earlier fitness methods.

The work of Dr. Dudley Sargent of Harvard, the man who believed in body measurements, was soon seen by others as too limiting. Fitness, they argued, was more than physique and stature. They began to establish performance parameters. Sargent himself joined this movement. From that time on, fitness was measured by how many pullups or situps you could do, how far you could broad-jump, how fast you could run.

But seconds on a stopwatch or numbers of repetitions are not equivalent to effort. They tell you nothing about the body's response to the exercise. They don't tell you if you're working hard enough, or not hard enough. There is only one way to tell whether you're working at the right intensity, and that is by measuring the amount of effort directly. No previous programs did this.

For years, Americans tried to keep themselves fit by practicing Walter Camp's Daily Dozen, a series of exercises this 1911 All-American used to keep in shape for football. The one great deficiency of the program was that you did the same thing all the time; it got increasingly easier and you wound up not getting a workout. Like the jogger who runs a mile every day in the same amount of time, the person on Walter Camp's program would be in worse shape at the end of the year than he was at the end of the second month.

Then came the isometric "dynamic tension" method of Charles Atlas, who won the title of the world's most perfectly developed man in 1921. This program, verified by Drs. Hettinger and Müller, suggested that you could take care of your exercise needs in six seconds every day. For skeletal-muscle fiber, that's true. But skeletal-muscle fiber isn't all there is to the body; its fitness doesn't define the fitness of the organism. An exercise that's all through in six seconds does nothing whatever for the cardiovascular system.

Next came the Royal Canadian Air Force Exercises. They were tremendously popular, and still are. They're better than nothing, but they leave much to be desired. Once again, the exercises are based on performance; they're not physiologically adjusted. They require you to increase the amount of work you do, but you never know if the physiological load is enough, or too much.

Then came Aerobics. Kenneth Cooper, who invented the system, recognized that Americans didn't need muscle strength. They needed endurance. But he neglected muscle altogether. He emphasized, instead, heart, circulation and oxygen consumption. All three are important considerations, but Cooper didn't provide a means to measure them. He simply made the assumption that the faster and farther you went, the more oxygen you would use. His thought was that if you just did all you could you would be sure to get trained.

Cooper's program came close to making the transition between external and internal control of exercise, but it didn't quite do the job. To equilibrate physical activity with oxygen consumption is full of errors. Why not go to the logical next step, and measure physiological response directly?

In the laboratory this can be done in many ways. We can measure how much oxygen you consume while you're working, how much air you're ventilating, how much your blood pressure is rising and how fast your pulse is beating. Of all these, pulse rate is the easiest to measure; it has the further advantage of computing the relative effort expended by various systems of the body and coming up with a final score, which is a reliable indicator of the intensity of physiological effort.

Now, for the first time, we could separate physical activity as a fitness event and physical activity as a sporting event. Where people seeking fitness had gotten hurt was in mingling the two. If you're jogging with another person with the objective of jogging farther than he can or faster than he can, then you're not jogging for fitness. And if you're unfit for this strenuous competition, it could be lethal.

From the standpoint of medical safety, the pulse-count system had compelling advantages over previous exercise systems. Yet it contained an inherent characteristic that caused doctors to get their backs up. The medical profession is invariably horrified at the thought that anyone but a doctor should do what doctors do. During World War II, physical-training personnel, encouraged by physical-education consultants, attempted to measure the response of recruits to exercise. One of the field tests was to measure the recovery rate of the heart. One day, a medical-corps colonel walking past the training field noticed that the physical-training instructors were using stethoscopes for fitness testing. "My God," he exploded, "what are those sergeants doing? Practicing medicine? Get those stethoscopes the hell out of there." Episodes like that one had discouraged me from considering the widespread use of pulse tests.

THE FIRST EXPERIMENTS WITH PULSE RATE

Experimentally, however, my work proceeded. During 1945 and 1946, I led an expedition for the National Academy of Sciences to determine the energy cost of military maneuvers in the snow. The United States was preparing for the possibility of war with the Soviet Union; any such war, it was thought, would be fought at least partially in Alaska. The government wanted to find out what it could expect of its soldiers in the snow. How much energy would they consume? How much food would they require? We conducted our experiments during maneuvers in New Hampshire. It was immediately apparent that heart rate or pulse count could be used to predict whether certain tasks could be performed. If we loaded a toboggan too heavily, or set too fast a speed, a soldier simply couldn't perform. His heart rate was simply too high. Not that the beat itself was too uncomfortable. It simply indicated that the subject was using energy too fast and would soon fatigue. Because we had deliberately chosen nonathletic subjects for our experiments, our findings could be translated to everyday use. A high pulse count for a sustained period signaled an inadequate capacity for the work

It wasn't for another fifteen years, however, that we were able to quantify pulse rate in relation to exercise. I was at that time on the academic committee of the National Research Council, working on the problem of turnaround times for ships. Our research site was San Francisco Harbor. One of the aspects to be studied was the work of longshoremen and stevedores. We wanted to measure the energy cost of their work. Such measurements are normally made in a laboratory, using mouthpieces, face masks and tanks on the back to collect expired air. I recommended that we use pulse rate to gauge the work levels of the various tasks. The results of the pulse test uncovered several bottlenecks. The men were working in hot, stuffy holds; as their temperatures rose and they perspired, their bodies began to store heat. The energy they should have been using to work was spent in perspiration. We found that we couldn't expect them to work continuously for more than half an hour when their pulse rate exceeded 150 beats a minute. If they worked at levels of 120 beats a minute, they could work for an hour or more. From these data and further studies, standards were set for the industry, and turnaround times improved.

From this experience, we were able, as well, to formulate a physiological work timetable for young, well-conditioned adults.

Pulse Rate	Industrial Work Times
Under 90	Above eight hours
90–110	Four to eight hours
110–130	One to four hours
130–150	Thirty to sixty minutes
150–170	One to thirty minutes
170–190	Thirty to sixty seconds
Above 190	Under thirty seconds

THE BREAKTHROUGH

Thus far, the use of the pulse-count method had been limited to academic pursuits.

Then two things happened that created an opportunity for much broader application. One was the creation of a highly specialized program for astronauts in prolonged space flights. The other, led by Dr. Fox, was the speculation that exercise might combat America's number-one killer, coronary heart disease. The two are wedded because the method to preserve the health and fitness of astronauts is directly applicable to preventive cardiology. In both cases it's highly important that the exercise be adequate to produce a conditioning stimulus and yet not so intensive that it might be damaging. To achieve that objective, in both cases, it was imperative to remove the emphasis on external performance—and place it, instead, on physiological exertion.

In 1964, Douglas Aircraft's space division asked

me to establish a bio-technology laboratory to develop techniques to preserve the health and fitness of astronauts in prolonged space-flight missions. My specific role was to define the needs for exercise and to develop instruments that could be used in zero gravity to measure the astronauts' response to exercise. The instruments were to have the double purpose of exercisers.

But what exercisers they would have to be! We weren't talking about just any ordinary fitness program. We were talking about men who would be spending two *years* in space. As I wrote out the requirements, I realized that if I gave the astronauts standard exercises to perform, and judged their condition by their response to this exercise, the program would fail. When you do an exercise repeatedly, you invariably approach it more comfortably and perform it in a more relaxed and skillful manner. This gives you a completely false response pattern. Because you're performing better, you get the impression that your physiological condition has improved. In reality, your condition would be deteriorating, because you're not getting a sufficient workout. What a disaster for the space program if the astronaut became so deconditioned —due not only to inactivity but to the reduced demands made on his system because of the lack of gravitational weight—that he couldn't accomplish what he'd been sent to do!

The answer was clear: I needed to approach the problem from inside the body rather than outside. By controlling the task, I would learn what the astronaut needed to put out in order to accomplish that task. The infallible index was his heart rate. If he could perform the task with ease, his heart rate would remain low. If he needed to exert, his heart rate would rise. If his heart rate remained low, he wasn't getting a stimulating workout. We could then elevate the stress in order to increase his heart rate.

It wasn't the outward physical performance we were after. It was the internal state of the astronauts that concerned us. We knew from the flights of Mercury and Gemini that physiological deterioration did occur, even in flights of two weeks' duration or less. We knew it would be important to detect this deterioration and correct it immediately if man was going to go on to the planets. Otherwise, he might be incapable of performing the necessary tasks to get there. His internal deterioration would creep up on him; suddenly, he'd be unable to do his work—and then it would be dangerously late to do anything about it.

I began to study this possibility. My studies led to my invention in 1966 of a physiologically adjusted "continuous environment regulator"—an elaborate stationary bicycle. The human body became, in effect, an automatic thermostat; its impulses were used to control the environment in which it existed. In the case of exercise, the heart rate during exercise automatically adjusted the resistance of the exerciser. A little computer in the mechanism sensed the difference between the desired heart rate and the actual heart rate. Every seven seconds, it made a calculation. Where a difference existed, the machine put more resistance on the pedals, so that the heart rate would rise to the desired level.

Two things were accomplished. Any time the medical monitor in Houston wanted to make an accurate assessment of any change in the function of the astronaut's cardiovascular system, he could compare the measurements on the test date with measurements of previous days and make a precise plot of where the astronaut was at that moment. In such fashion, the monitor could prescribe what the astronaut needed to do in order to get where he ought to be. The second advantage was that the astronaut could exercise at the prescribed heart rate each day. The importance of this can be appreciated only when we compare our situation to that of the astronauts. We have gravity, which exercises us automatically; our muscles must constantly push against it every time we move. A few minutes a day of concentrated exercise keeps us in shape. The astronauts have no gravity whatever; they get no postural exercise at all. Accordingly, they must exercise ninety minutes a day during prolonged space flights in order to remain in adequate shape to perform the tasks of their mission.

THE ASTRONAUTS' PROGRAM AND YOU

But if our circumstances are different from those of the astronauts, the need for exercise is the same. In each case, a certain amount of extra physical activity must be performed in order to remain fit.

And the method used by the astronauts to make certain they get just enough exercise—no more, no less—worked just as well on earth. By exercising at a specific heart-rate level, the astronauts—or anyone—could maintain the body's condition at the desired level. Any change from day to day in physiological status would automatically become part of the consideration in determining how much physical work you have to do. When you're fatigued or not feeling well, your heart rate responds more swiftly to stress; the weaker you are, the less work required to get your heart rate up.

In the old way of exercising, you had to perform a certain task a certain number of times. It made no allowance for the condition of your system at the moment you performed the exercise. The new way automatically compensates for your condition by using your very own computer. On days when you're not feeling well, it takes less work to obtain the desired heart rate or level of physiological activity. So if your program is to maintain a heartbeat of 130 for five minutes, you're always giving the same effort for that exercise. If you're fatigued, then you have to put out less work to reach the same effort level. As training takes place, then you have to do more work to produce the same effort.

The lay person uses "effort" and "work" synonymously. The physiologist doesn't. Effort is the energy you expend. Work is the physical action that effort produces. Physical work is calculated by measuring force and displacement. Physiological effort is a man's reaction during physical activity in terms of his internal functions: metabolism, respiration and circulation. When you're bicycling, I can see how much work you're doing, but I don't know how much effort you're expending to accomplish the work. When I look at a heart meter or check your pulse rate, I see how much effort you're expending, but I don't know how much work that effort is accomplishing. In a fitness program, I don't even *care* how much work you're accomplishing; all that concerns me is your heart rate. If you're exercising on a hot day, your body will store heat and you'll be adding the effort to lose this heat on top of your exertion to keep exercising. Your internal computer adds these two requirements. So, to maintain your desired heart rate on a hot day would accomplish very little physically, but you would have an adequate fitness workout. (Not as desirable, however, as if your body had remained cool. Remember that when you don't get the support from those auxiliary hearts, your skeletal muscles, your heart is on its own in moving the blood around.)

The lessons I had learned while developing techniques to preserve the astronauts' health and fitness soon found broader application. The call from Dr. Fox of the U.S. Public Health Service came in the midst of my work. I was convinced that what the astronauts did to remain fit could be used by earthlings to prevent heart disease.

The program I developed at the instigation of the U.S. Public Health Service has found numbers of devotees since that time. They include sheriffs, firemen and lifeguards of Los Angeles County, YMCA's throughout the United States, and housewives across the country who use the program to keep their health—and their figures.

They all know that it's not the physical performance that's important, it's the exertion it takes to perform. Their purpose is not to beat some other person, or lift some heavier weight, or run faster than they ever have. It's to get their bodies fit. They properly keep their minds not on the external result, but on the internal mechanism.

If your goal is to have a better-functioning internal organism—better heart, lungs, and blood vessels, firmer bones, stronger muscles—then that's what you focus your attention on, not on how much weight these bones and muscles can lift or how far the heart and the muscles can run. Unless you're an athlete, who cares if you can run fast? The important thing is to have a better internal mechanism, a better-quality body to help you live a life filled with days of feeling good.

Until this moment, all physical conditioning has been based on external performance. It's time to get under the skin.

VII

All About Your Pulse

The pulse is a wave initiated by the heart. It travels throughout your arterial system each time your heart beats.

It's the change in the condition of your artery at the end of each heartbeat, at the point at which you feel the change.

In most people, the pulse can be felt wherever a large artery lies near the surface—at the temple, in the throat, at the wrist, inside the thigh, on top. of the foot.

If you put one hand over your heart and then feel the pulse of that hand with your other hand, you'll notice a little lag in time between the beats. The heart has finished beating before you feel the pulse in your wrist. This is because the change in the artery is like the change in a garden hose when someone runs over it with a car. As the heart beats and the valves close, a wave of change travels down from the artery to your wrist. You can duplicate this effect by holding a garden hose near the nozzle in one hand with the water on, then stamping on the hose near the faucet with your foot. It will take a moment for you to feel the hose "pulse." If you press on the hose quickly and then release, and repeat the movement once a second, the hand holding the hose near the nozzle will feel each one of these kicks, but there will be a lag time, depending on the length of the hose. If you kick five times, you'll eventually feel five changes. Your action will make practically no change in the flow of water. The water pressure will drop off just a bit, but the total flow will remain almost constant.

The rate at which these pulses occur will not tell you how much water is going through the hose, nor will it give you an index of water pressure. Similarly, when you read a pulse, you're not reading the amount of blood flowing out of the heart into the body, nor are you reading blood pressure. The pulse is nothing more or less than an accurate index of how many times the heart is beating against the column of blood in your circulatory vessels.

But what a wonderful index it is! It informs you of every change that is taking place in your person. It tells you if your body temperature is rising, or if you're cooling down. It tells you how fast you're burning up energy and using oxygen from the air. It tells you how your body is handling the chemical wastes in your blood. It tells you how your muscles are involved and working. It even tells you about the state of your emotions and attitudes. It pulls all of these things together, weighs them and comes out with a single signal that reports your overall condition.

The pulse is so simple to measure, and yet it's

the body's most important single indicator of well-being, stress or illness.

Not only is the pulse a simple and reliable index, it's easy to locate and count. After light exercise, it's impossible to miss. After moderate exercise, you don't even have to search for it. If you just sit quietly, you can feel it beating.

You can find your pulse by putting your hand over your heart, by feeling the pulse in your wrist, or by just sitting quietly and listening. You can also feel it in the carotid artery at the side of your neck. If you use this method, be sure not to try to feel the two arteries at either side of the neck at the same time. This is the sole route of blood to the brain. If you press on both sides at once, you're diminishing the blood flow or cutting it off entirely.

Some people can feel their pulse in the temporal arteries next to the ear. Some can even feel it in the thumb—which is the reason you don't use your thumb for counting pulse. If you use your thumb to take someone else's pulse, you might be feeling your pulse, and miss the other person's entirely.

Your pulse rate changes throughout the day. It is lowest after you have been asleep about six hours. On awakening it will increase five to ten beats per minute. During the day your resting pulse rate gradually increases, and at bedtime it is probably another five to ten beats per minute higher than it was when you got up in the morning. Any activity, such as eating, elevates the pulse rate. A bout of hard work such as heavy gardening can cause the pulse rate to be elevated for the rest of the day, and most of the night.

WHAT YOUR PULSE TELLS YOU ABOUT FITNESS

The relation of pulse to fitness is hardly a new topic. Huang Ti, the "Yellow Emperor of China," who lived from 2697 B.C. to 2597 B.C., declared: "The heart is in accord with the pulse." Plutarch wrote in *Moralia: Advice about Keeping Well:* "Each person ought neither to be unacquainted with the peculiarities of his own pulse, for there are many individual diversities."

There are four things you can feel when sensing your pulse. The first is the force of the pulse against your fingers. As you become fit, this force gets stronger. The second is the volume, or expansion of the artery. As you become fit, the volume increases, and the artery feels thicker, yet soft and elastic. The third is the regularity of the force and the rhythm. As you become fit, your pulse becomes stronger and more regular. The fourth is the frequency. As you become fit, the frequency of pulse beats diminishes.

Lower pulse is an advantage because it indicates that the heart is taking a longer period of rest between beats, meaning that it fills more slowly and completely. There is twice the filling time at a heart rate of sixty beats a minute as there is at ninety beats a minute. This increase in pumping efficiency results in an improved supply of oxygen to the heart, and improved coronary blood flow. When you realize that the average coronary volume per heartbeat—the amount going into the circulation that nourishes the heart—is only one teaspoon of blood, the importance of blood flow becomes apparent.

Your resting pulse rate while seated gives you important information about your health and fitness. Men average 72 to 76 beats a minute, boys 80 to 84 beats a minute. Women average 75 to 80 beats a minute, girls 82 to 89 beats a minute. The reason why women and girls have slightly higher pulse rates than men and boys isn't understood.

Rates as low as 50 and as high as 100 can still be within the normal range, according to the American Heart Association. The U.S. Air Force has found some normal cadets with heart rates as low as 30 beats a minute, and as high as 110. But in general, the lower the resting heart rate, the healthier you are. Resting heart rates higher than 80 beats a minute are suggestive of poor health and fitness, an increased risk of coronary heart disease and death in middle age. The mortality rate for men and women with pulse rates over 92 is four times greater than for those with pulse rates less than 67.

An accelerated pulse rate in itself isn't dangerous. Nor does it indicate that there's something necessarily wrong with you. All it means is that the body is working under a heavy load. A pulse rate above 120 borders on intensive exertion. The efficiency of the body is measured by how much external work is being accomplished at a moderate heart rate of about 120. If it takes very little physical work to produce this kind of heart rate, that means you're "inefficient." Your system is probably deconditioned due to lack of exercise.

The following table will indicate the approximate pulse rates that are reached at various intensities of continuous exercise.

Scale of Perceived Exertion	Pulse Rate
1—Very, very light	Under 90
2—Very light	90
3—Light	100
4—Fairly light	110
5—Neither light nor heavy ("moderate")	120
6—Somewhat heavy	130
7—Heavy	140
8—Very heavy	150
9—Very, very heavy	160

Pulse rate is affected by emotion as well as exertion. Such influence is on the side of safety in exercise. An athlete playing in an important game will have a pulse rate so elevated that he will appear to be playing harder than he actually is. But fitness exercises do not have a high emotional component, so the exercise pulse is a reliable guide to the intensity of the effort.

Your exercise pulse rate is quite independent of your resting rate. Once you start exercising, your rate will be elevated in accordance with the intensity of the exercise. Whether your resting rate was 60 or 80, moderate exercise will raise your pulse rate to about 120.

If your pulse rate is racing at 100 or 110 while you're sitting, your heart is working as it would be if you were walking. But you're at a disadvantage because of the lack of action of your leg muscles to keep the blood flowing. The heart is doing it all—and that's a strain.

If your pulse rate is over 100 beats a minute, this could indicate that you've had previous physical activity, or that your body is not in a resting state even though you may be sitting down, or that you may have been stimulated by coffee or cigarettes —both caffeine and nicotine raise heart and pulse rate by as much as ten beats a minute—or that you have a slight fever. If it isn't any of these things, then you have an extraordinarily high resting heart rate, a condition known as tachycardia. If your heart rate is at the upper limits of the scale of normal, near 100 beats a minute, it's mandatory that you attempt to lower the rate—with your physician's help —if it's over 100. A high resting rate is inefficient and tiring. The heart is working harder than it should be.

Even if your heart rate is at the lower limits of normal, you'll do well to lower it still further. A slow heart beats more efficiently. There's no danger in lowering your heart rate, no matter how low you are to begin with.

WHY EXERCISE LOWERS THE HEART RATE

The best way yet discovered to lower the resting heart rate is, paradoxically, to make it beat faster during prolonged periods of exercise. This exertion strengthens the heart so that it performs more efficiently at lower rates. This lowered heart rate is called the "bradycardia" of training.

Marathon runners and other endurance athletes characteristically have low heart or pulse rates.

Heart rates below 40 have been recorded in superior athletes. A heart rate below 40 is usually suspected to be a pathological condition caused by a conduction disturbance in which the nerve impulses have difficulty passing through the tissues of the heart. I remember one athlete who stunned an examining physician and a consulting cardiologist when they found his pulse rate to be only 34 beats a minute. At first they wouldn't let him exercise. But after careful study of the athlete under laboratory conditions, they decided that an extremely low heart rate was perfectly healthy for him.

The heart is strengthened two ways during exercise, first by improving the quality of the heart muscle, called the myocardium, and second by increasing the coordination of the fibers as they wring blood out of the heart during each beat. The heart works something like a wet towel when you wring the water out of it. To demonstrate the action, once again put the fingers of the left hand into the palm of the right hand, and squeeze those fingers with the right hand, just as the muscles of the heart squeeze against the blood. If all the fingers squeeze together with the same amount of force, the fingers of your other hand will be tightly compressed. If the fingers squeeze weakly and out of concert, the compression won't be nearly as forceful. Each squeezing finger represents a group of heart fibers. If they all move in a continuous, rhythmic manner, then each set of fibers has less work to do. The fibers are like athletes: they need training. When they're unused, they're uncoordinated. Some of the fibers become lazy, so others have to work harder and more frequently in order to move the blood around in required quantities.

In exercise, you have an increased return of blood from the veins, which gives the heart resistance to beat against. It's the resistance, or loading, that causes the heart to develop.

The heart too needs its "overload" if it is to be conditioned. To achieve this "overload," you must pursue an activity that pushes your heart rate to a level a little higher than you get in everyday routine activities. Your goal is to eventually get your pulse up to 120 and hold it there for a few minutes —every day, if possible. Milder exercise is better than nothing, but not sufficient to increase your heart's vigor.

The purpose of the heart is to pump blood from the venous system into the arterial system. The total output of that pump is called cardiac output. It's measured in volume of blood per minute. Your heart rate is the main means by which you increase the circulation of blood. From low heart rates to intermediate heart rates, the heart is able to increase the circulation by increasing the stroke volume—the amount of blood ejected by the heart into the arterial system each time the heart beats. Up to 110 beats a minute, you're getting a strong assist from the stroke-volume increase. After 110, this influence is less and less. After 130, if you're not in good shape, the circulation is increased by heart rate alone. At a heart rate of 130 or higher, the heart is beating so fast that it doesn't have time to fill any greater volume, so the amount of blood the heart puts out varies in direct proportion to the number of beats per minute. It's a lot more efficient for the heart to have both systems, the stroke-volume increases and the pulse-rate increases, working to increase its output.

Now the effects of conditioning become apparent. If you're well conditioned, you can extend this contribution of stroke volume up to 140 beats a minute because of the more efficient coordination of the fibers of the heart. If the heart is in poor condition, then stroke-volume contribution may quit at 120 beats a minute.

Beyond 170 to 180 beats a minute, cardiac output doesn't increase even if your heart beats faster. You've reached the limit of venous return to the heart.

The heart may go above 200 beats a minute. Heartbeats as high as 230 have been recorded during exercise. Each person has his own maximum. It's not important that you can get your heart rate up to 220 and I can get mine only to 210 or that someone else can get his only to 190. Many top athletes can't get their heart rates above 190. Maximum heart rate is not an index of physical fitness. Long-term training may have no effect at all on increasing your maximum heart rate. Maximum heart rate lowers as you age; studies of a large population in Sweden have demonstrated that the average maximum heart rate drops about one beat per minute each year. The reason why it decreases with age isn't well understood, but it has no bearing on your capacity to function, in any case.

For large adult populations, the average maximum heart rate is approximately 220 beats a minute minus the person's age. This isn't an ideal figure, or a goal, or one to put into competition. It's a theoretical estimate of maximum exercise pulse rate at various ages.

HOW TO LOWER YOUR RESTING HEART RATE USING THE PULSE-COUNT GUIDE

You don't have to be a marathon runner to lower your resting heart rate about ten beats a minute. Any training you do that puts a slight overload on your heart will do the job. If you're untrained, the amount of exertion you would need to expend would be relatively slight. You might even accomplish it by walking.

If your heart rate is low to begin with, this doesn't mean that you've got the endurance to go out and race two miles. You have to prepare your heart just as carefully as does the man whose heart rate is high at the outset of his program.

When we come to the exercise program, we'll give you a formula to calculate your pulse count during each of its phases. For the moment, let's establish some parameters.

At the outset of your program, you'll exercise at 150 minus your age, at a minimum. Thus, if you are fifty years old and just starting out on a fitness program, you will exercise at 100 beats a minute. If you're fifty and you've been working out for a few months, or are in pretty fair shape to begin with, you can exercise at a rate of 170 minus your age, or 120. If you are in excellent condition at the age of fifty and wish to exercise vigorously, you can work at 190 minus your age, or 140.

The harder you work, the better it will be—to a point. One hundred ten is a great deal better than 100. But 150 is only a tiny bit better than 140. No further health benefits for the heart can be obtained by increasing the rate above 200 minus your age.

As your condition improves, it's important that you work out at around 120. The well-conditioned person will not improve anything if he works below 120.

You can get good results within a month. If your resting heart rate is 95 at the beginning of training, it should be 90 after a month of training. If your heart rate hasn't lowered, you should increase the quantity of cardio-respiratory endurance exercise.

Your maximum heart rate may be higher initially than that of an athlete. Your minimum may be lower than that of an athlete. These highs and lows are not predictive of your physical performance. Where you are to begin with is not important. It's how you lower your rate in training that's important. A primary goal of your training will be to lower your resting heart rate five to ten beats a minute *regardless* of what it was at the outset.

This lowered heart rate is the barometer of the relaxed power that you see in highly trained athletes and sleek wild animals. It is the characteristic of a well-trained person—one who has so much power available that he can perform with ease, who feels more alive, less fatigued, with an almost unlimited capacity for activity.

VIII

Your Pulse Test

It's time to get fit.

Before anything, we have to make certain that your present condition is such that you can undertake a fitness program without endangering your health.

The best assurance, of course, is from your doctor. If you've had a medical checkup within the last year, the chances are that you can start your program. Had your doctor found some reason why you shouldn't engage in moderate exercise, he would surely have told you at the time. Nonetheless, it would be a good idea to call him now and make certain you can proceed.

If you've developed any of the following symptoms after hurrying up a flight of stairs or carrying a bag down an airport ramp or engaging in mild exercise such as gardening, you should see your doctor immediately—and you should definitely not undertake a program until you do.

Pains in the chest
Dizziness or faintness
Gastrointestinal upset
Difficulty in breathing
Flu-like symptoms

One simple measure of whether you are fit enough to engage in moderate exercise is your ability to walk two miles. If you can't do that, it's as specific a warning as one from your doctor—and you should see him about it.

I'm not trying to scare you. I simply want you to be prudent. If you're severely deconditioned, there are certain combinations you have to avoid that are formulas for physiological disaster. If you're an overeater who stuffs himself with food until he feels uncomfortable, you're primed for trouble. If you overdrink *and* overeat at the same time (as is usually the case), one further increment could kill you. It could be a hot bath. It could be a strained bowel movement. Or it could be a bout of exercise.

It goes without saying that if you're about to have a heart attack, you shouldn't exercise. The person described above is a candidate for one. There are other contraindications to exercise: inflammations, fevers, or respiratory problems, like pulmonary edema. Athletes can compete when they have a cold or a fever. The rest of us should skip it. We're not competing with anyone.

If any of the following categories applies to you, be sure to check with your doctor before starting the program:

High blood pressure
Heavy smoking
High cholesterol
Total lack of exercise
History of heart disease in your immediate family
Tension
Obesity

One further injunction against an exercise program at this time is if over thirty percent of your body is fat. That's the medical definition of obesity. You don't need a laboratory test to tell you if you're obese; you can see the fat hanging from your body in pendulous folds. If that's your condition, you should lose weight under medical supervision before you start any intensive exercise. What you can do in addition is to begin a moderate walking program as a preliminary to the fitness program you'll undertake when you've lost some weight.

Even if you've seen your doctor recently, and he's cleared you for exercise, there's an additional test to be made before you begin your program. Your doctor almost always sees you in a state of rest. Most office examinations don't include an exercise electrocardiogram on a stepping bench, treadmill or bicycle ergometer. Consequently, when you start your program you need to watch for signs of poor tolerance that would show up only when you exercise.

You administer this test yourself, by counting your pulse in various conditions of rest and mild exercise. Physical exercise should feel good; there should be absolutely no feeling of discomfort; this test is to make certain there won't be.

The test will be no harder than climbing stairs. It consists of taking your pulse while you sit, then stand and finally step up and down for three one-minute periods. I'll tell you what to look for to see that you are responding well to these exertions. The results will make certain that it's safe for you to begin increasing your physical capacity on your own under my guidance.

For the test, you'll need a wristwatch or a clock with a sweep second hand. You'll also need a ruler, to measure the height of the step you'll be using during your test.

HOW TO COUNT YOUR PULSE RATE

First, you'll want to find the best place to feel your pulse. Be active for a minute or so in any manner you wish—take a brisk walk, or climb a flight of stairs—in order to amplify your pulse. Now explore the following:

The radial artery in your wrist, just inside your wrist bone at the base of your thumb joint.

A carotid artery on one side of your throat, either just above your collarbone or below your jaw. Remember, don't close off the second carotid artery on the other side while you're doing this; you may shut down the blood supply to your brain.

A temporal artery at the side of your forehead

(temple) just in front of your ear. Again, press on one side *only*.

Most people prefer the radial artery in the wrist. If that's the system you elect, use the following procedure:

Place your wristwatch on your wrist so that you can see its face when the palm of your hand is up. Next, place the wrist on which you have your watch in the palm of your other hand, so that the wrist falls into the crotch between thumb and forefinger. Let the tips of your fingers curl toward your thumb. Now your third and fourth fingers will rest over your pulse. The little pads at the ends of those fingers will fit right into the groove of the wrist. The pad on your middle finger is the pulse "feeler." If you press slightly against the wrist with your fingertip feeler, you should be able to find your pulse. Don't panic if you can't find the pulse at first; it takes a few minutes of practice.

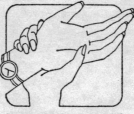

TAKING YOUR PULSE

What you feel at each beat is not blood flow, but a pulse wave that moves along the arteries about twelve to eighteen feet per second.

Doctors and nurses use one of several methods

in taking the pulse: counting it for a minute, counting it for thirty seconds and multiplying by two, or counting for fifteen seconds and multiplying by four. We use still another method: counting for six seconds and adding a zero. We do this for a good reason. A longer count is more accurate in general terms and is ideal for taking the pulse of someone at rest. But a long count does not tell us about your exercise response as accurately as does a six-second count taken immediately after the exercise. Then the pulse (and heart) is beating at a rate that most nearly reflects the exertion you achieved during your movements. Within fifteen seconds, the pulse has diminished from that peak, within thirty seconds still more, and within a minute still more. The variation between the pulse rate immediately after exercise and the rate one minute later can be as much as thirty beats.

You're now going to determine your pulse rate by counting the number of pulses in six seconds and adding a zero to get the per-minute rate. Catch the rhythm of pulsations for a while. When your pulse coincides with an easy time interval (at one of the five-second marks) start counting. Begin with "Zero" as the second hand crosses over the five-second mark. If you don't say "Zero" you'll miscalculate. Then count the number of pulses in six seconds.

TAKING THE TEST

The test has six grades.

Grade One is to record and interpret your pulse at rest. Grade Two is to do the same when you're standing. Grades Three, Four and Five determine your reaction to mild exertion. Grade Six tests your rate of recovery.

It's best to take the test a few hours after eating, smoking or drinking. All three will elevate your pulse. Coffee is to be particularly avoided.

If you've been physically active, rest for a few minutes before starting, so that your pulse has a chance to become steady at a low level.

You shouldn't talk to anyone during the test, because conversation increases the pulse rate. If you want to experiment, take your pulse, then count out loud to ten or talk to someone, and then take your pulse again. Your resting rate will now probably be ten beats a minute higher than before.

If you're shivery or overheated, you'll get a false resting pulse rate as well. Either condition accelerates the pulse rate.

Once you're seated and calm, repeated counts will give about the same score. This score represents your usual resting heart rate during a day. The only time you would find your *basal* pulse would be on awakening in the morning and before you had left your bed. The resting rate while seated comes closer to the normal condition of wakefulness.

If during the test you have to clear your throat or cough, or you happen to yawn, wait a few minutes and start over. A fit of coughing, for example, can raise your heart rate twenty to thirty beats a minute. If you breathe deeply or forcibly, your pulse will speed up and slow down in rhythm with your respiration. While you are quiet and breathing softly your pulse should have a regular rhythm. (If it is irregular—if you feel a missed beat or an extra beat once in a while—tell your physician about it before you step up your physical activity.)

When you think you have a steady resting pulse rate, try a series of "biofeedback exercises" that can deliberately slow your pulse rate by releasing a lot of the excess tension in your body. Instead of sitting on a chair, let yourself sit *into* the chair. Let all your weight go into the chair. Instead of holding your legs up off the floor, let the weight of your legs move into your feet so that your feet feel heavy on the floor. Now let your shoulders drop comfortably outward instead of holding them up. Let your face relax; feel that you are no longer furrowing your forehead, squinting your eyes or clenching your teeth. Finally, let your belly relax. Put your hands on your belly. Do they rise or fall as you take a breath? In two out of every five cases I have examined, the belly is drawn in as breath is drawn in. This is backward breathing. Your abdomen is moving in opposition to your respiration. You're creating excess tension. Try to reverse the pattern. As you take in a breath, let your hands move outward.

Now take your pulse again. If you've done all of the above properly, your pulse should be measurably lower.

In this relaxed, quiet state, you're going to register your lowest seated pulse rate. It should be less than 100 beats per minute. If your seated pulse rate is near ten counts in six seconds, you'd better remain seated and get a full minute count. If it's 100 or over, try some more biofeedback relaxation to see if you can bring it down. If your pulse remains at 100 or more, you may have a fever or an infection. If this is the case, you shouldn't continue with the pulse fitness test until your illness has disappeared.

But if you don't have a fever and can't explain why your pulse is higher than 100, then it's prudent to check with your doctor to be sure that the rapid pulse is normal for you and that there is no reason why you shouldn't go ahead with activity.

If your pulse rate is less than 100—ten beats in six seconds—you may proceed to Grade Two.

GRADE TWO: ORTHOSTATIC TOLERANCE

Now we're going to test another aspect of your response to exercise—your orthostatic tolerance. This is the ability of your circulatory system to adjust to the vertical position after you have been sitting for a while.

Stand quietly for one minute. Remain in an easy resting position, not rigidly at attention. Shift your weight or wiggle your toes, as you wish, but don't move around. At the end of a minute, count your pulse. The difference between your sitting pulse rate and your standing pulse rate is another key indicator of your present level of fitness. If your standing pulse rate is twenty beats or more higher than your sitting pulse rate, that's probably higher than it should be, so ask your doctor if it means anything that would contraindicate increased physical exertion. If your pulse rate has gone up to 11 or more in six seconds, that's 110 per minute, or if you feel faint or dizzy your doctor should know about it, as there may be some significant reason for this poor orthostatic tolerance. Athletic ability doesn't enhance your ability to stand quietly. Top athletes faint as readily as sedentary people. An exercise program doesn't increase one's tolerance to quiet standing.

Your pulse rate *should* go up some; up to ten beats a minute is okay. In our system, if your sitting rate was 7 and your standing rate was 8, you're fit to proceed to Grade Three. Any change of one count in six seconds is okay—provided you don't hit 11.

GRADES THREE THROUGH SIX

Grade Three is the first of three one-minute exercises on a step. You'll want to measure the height of the step with a ruler, and consult the accompanying table. Find your body weight and move laterally across the table to where it intersects with the vertical column for your height step. Example: A woman weighing 140 pounds using an eight-inch step will step at a rate of thirty lifts per minute.

Stepping Rate (steps per minute)

Height of Step (inches)

		7	8	9	10	11	12
	100	30	30	30	30	30	30
	120	30	30	30	30	30	30
	140	30	30	30	30	20	20
	160	30	30	30	20	20	20
Body Weight (Pounds)	180	30	30	20	20	20	20
	200	30	20	20	20	20	20
	220	20	20	20	20	20	20

The test is simple: Step up with your left foot, then your right foot. Step down with your left foot, then your right foot. Repeat the lifts as many times as indicated on the table. Try to finish in one minute, no faster or no slower. You can tell after fifteen seconds whether your rhythm is sufficient to achieve the required number of steps. If you're going too fast or too slow, adjust accordingly.

Stop the test exercise at the first sign of poor tolerance.

There are several possible symptoms of poor tolerance. The first would be your attitude: you felt like quitting, you wanted to slow down, you ran out of gas, you began to feel worn out. Physical indications would be profuse sweat, cramps, achy legs, a tremor or twitching in the legs, shortness of breath, difficulty in breathing, a pounding heart that hurts. *Any* of these symptoms in a minute of mild exercise is a signal to stop your test and seek medical advice. If you stop, sit down. Don't ever stand quietly after exercise.

The moment you finish, sit down and count your pulse. If you felt some distress, or your count is 12 or more, your test is over and you have ascertained that you have a low tolerance to exercise. This probably means that you are deconditioned and are in need of an exercise program, but before you continue, talk it over with your physician.

If you experience none of the symptoms of poor tolerance and your count in six seconds is below 12, proceed to Grade Four. Repeat the one-minute test exercise immediately. Then sit and count your pulse. If it's 12 or more in six seconds, stop. If it's under 12, proceed to Grade Five. Once again, repeat immediately. Take your pulse. The standards are identical to Grades Three and Four. So are the admonitions.

Grade Six tests your recovery rate.

As soon as you complete Grade Five, sit down, take your pulse, rest for a minute and take your pulse again. Your pulse rate one minute after the exercise should fall at least ten beats per minute. The rate should be no more than 110 beats a minute.

RESULTS

If it took very little activity to get your pulse to 120, then you're in poor condition. But if your heart rate didn't pass 120 after the three stepping exercises and you were comfortable throughout, then you're in pretty good shape.

This pulse test works well for our purposes. It's not a medical test. It doesn't diagnose anything. What it does is turn up any sign of poor tolerance you may not have noticed before, and it shows you what your level of fitness for exercise is at the present time.

If you stopped the test before Grade Three, get a medical okay before you exercise further.

If your pulse went above 120 beats per minute in Grade Three, start your fitness exercise program at Training Pulse Rate 1 (TPR-1).

If your pulse went above 120 in Grade Four, start your program at TPR-2.

If your pulse went above 120 in Grade Five, start your program at TPR-3.

If you went through all six grades, if your pulse did not exceed 120 beats per minute, and if your pulse one minute after exercise fell more than ten beats per minute, you can begin the fitness exercise program at TPR-4.

The Training Pulse Rate chart is found on page 209.

Whether you start at TPR-1 or TPR-4, your program will consist of three simple exercises you'll perform ten minutes a day, three times a week. Before we come to these exercises, however, let's consider how you can keep your present condition and avoid further deterioration without any exercise at all.

THE PULSE TEST

Grade One: Record pulse at rest	If count is under 100, go on to Grade Two
Grade Two: Record pulse standing up	If change is less than ten beats per minute, and you feel okay, go on to Grade Three
Grade Three: Step exercise one minute	If count is under 120, and you feel okay, go on to Grade Four
Grade Four: Repeat exercise	If count is under 120, and you feel okay, go on to Grade Five
Grade Five: Repeat exercise	
Grade Six: Sit quickly and count pulse immediately After one minute of rest, count pulse again	

Results:

a) If you went through six grades, if your pulse did not exceed 120 beats per minute, and if your pulse after one minute of rest fell more than ten beats per minute, you can begin the fitness exercise program at TPR-4 (See pages 208-09).

b) If your pulse went above 120 in Grade Five, start the program at TPR-3.

c) If your pulse went above 120 in Grade Four, start the program at TPR-2.

d) If your pulse went above 120 in Grade Three, start the program at TPR-1.

e) If you stopped the test before Grade Three, get a medical okay before you exercise further.

IX

Minimum Maintenance

When I was chief of performance physiology for the Air Force in the late forties, my department was asked to find out why air-transport pilots, as a group, did not live as long as other personnel, and had the shortest active careers of any occupation in the United States. The speculation was that their erosion had to do with vibration, noxious gases in the cockpits, prolonged low levels of oxygen or just plain fear of flying. Our studies determined that it was none of these. Rather, it was what the pilots did when they finished flying. Their flights would put them down at lonely bases near isolated towns. Invariably, they would repair to a bar, get loaded, eat a fat steak and spend the night partying with a date.

That's an extreme case of what confronts all of us to a degree. Tension, boredom and fatigue drive us to seek release. We reward ourselves with lazy hours and as much luxury as we can afford. Advertisers orient our instincts, cheer us on and soothe our consciences. The consequences are devastating.

Much of the human deterioration that we attribute to aging is simply a manifestation of deconditioning caused by inactivity. The feeble, slouching, uncoordinated person who stumbles past us may be in early middle age.

Consider Bob P., who played Ivy League football in the fifties and then became a stockbroker. The day he walked off the playing field, he vowed that he would never run again unless he had to to save his life. He was only half joking. Today, he's a fitness mess. A flight of stairs might as well be a mountain. Windows are harder to raise. A jar of peanuts finally threw him; he couldn't get it open.

Bob recognized that he was no longer master of his environment, and determined to do something about it. The results were tragicomic. First he went to a commercial gym, but found that he couldn't keep up with the weight lifters. Moreover, he was uncomfortable being around them and embarrassed to undress in front of them. Then he went to the local high-school track and couldn't jog more than a few hundred yards. The physical pain didn't hurt nearly as much as the knowledge that twenty years before he had sprinted around just such an oval. Finally, Bob turned to sports. It was his worst mistake. Two sets left him with tennis elbow. An hour of touch football left him immobile for a week. He was fortunate. Either contest could have killed him.

You don't turn to sports to get fit. The man who suddenly determines to get back into shape should not look around for a tennis partner. Competition creates stress—and just that amount of stress for a burdened man who is out of shape could be lethal.

A few years ago, I gave a quiz to directors of health-club programs. Several of the questions pertained to the relationship between exercise and stress. The fitness leaders—most of whose work is with aging men—agreed for the most part that exercise was always excellent therapy for stress. They were wrong.

If you're under severe emotional stress you shouldn't exercise. You've had your workout for that day. By severe stress, I mean when you're wrung out emotionally, when someone you cared for has died, or when you've just been fired. That's no time to add one stress to another.

Exercise can be therapeutic, however, for the person undergoing normal stress. Physical exercise reorganizes the functions of the body. When you're harassed and frustrated, you actually feel as though little pieces of you are lying all about. That's because the controlling systems of the body, the autonomic nervous system and the sympathetic nervous system, fail to control function in a harmonious way. Physical exercise picks up these pieces and puts them back together again by putting an organized demand on the body that brings these control systems into play.

If you have let your physical condition deteriorate, the chances are that you are either unfit or at best only moderately fit for sport. This doesn't mean that you shouldn't play the sport while you're getting yourself back into shape. It means that you should be extremely careful how you go about it. You should choose an opponent who is in approximately the same condition. You shouldn't get overzealous. And you shouldn't confuse what you're doing with a true fitness program.

In order to have a fitness program, you must first determine how fit you want to be.

If your objective is to maintain your present level of fitness and prevent deterioration, you don't require any special exercises. You can incorporate a fitness program into your everyday routine. For example, you can maintain your present muscle tone by lifting a small child once a day. Assuming there's a small child handy, what could be simpler? A few bags of heavy groceries will achieve the same result. This load on your muscles provides them with "minimum maintenance." Let's put that term into context.

There are three levels of satisfactory fitness. The first is the irreducible minimum below which you're going to experience degradation of function and structure. The second is a general level of fitness that provides you with a safe margin of adaptation for change, including emergencies, and enables you to get through the day without an undue amount of fatigue. The third level is preparation for fairly strenuous recreational or occupational activity.

The third level requires specific conditioning. If you're going skiing you've got to do pre-skiing exercises or you just won't ski as well. The second level, general fitness, requires the thirty-minute-a-week program we'll detail in Chapters X and XI. The first level, minimum maintenance, requires nothing more than the incorporation of a few simple habits into everyday life.

Whether you want to be a superathlete or a well-conditioned person, you must still adopt these few basic habits for everyday life. In order to reach level two or three, in other words, you've got to pass level one.

THE FIVE REQUIREMENTS
OF MAINTENANCE

Minimum maintenance can be achieved by meeting five simple requirements every day:

1. Limber up by reaching arms, twisting trunk, bending waist and turning trunk.

2. Stand for a total of two hours during the day.

3. Lift something unusually heavy for five seconds.

4. Walk briskly for at least three minutes to stimulate your cardiovascular system.

5. Burn up three hundred calories a day in physical activity. (See calorie chart, page 182.)

All five requirements can be met with ease.

Shopping for groceries takes care of three and possibly four of the five requirements, with just a touch of emphasis on your part. Consider the first requirement, to work the body's joints. Instead of turning around when you're looking for something, *twist* around. Bend for groceries on the bottom shelf. Stretch for them on the top shelf. That's your mobility exercise for the day.

Shopping takes anywhere up to an hour. That's half your standing requirement for the day. The other half is compiled when you shower, shave, make your bed, do the dishes, stand at someone's desk and so on.

There are two reasons for standing. The first is to condition yourself for orthostatic tolerance—which means to keep from fainting when you stand up. When you're lying down or sitting, gravity is just pulling a short distance; it's easy for the blood to flow. When you move to a vertical position, the whole column of blood stands on end. Now it's difficult for the blood in the veins to get back to the heart. By standing frequently during the day, you condition the vessels to constrict the lower parts of your body so the blood doesn't pool in your ankles. Now the blood can be returned to the heart, and from there be pumped to the brain. The second reason for standing frequently is to put a longitudinal stress on the bones. For some reason we don't understand, this type of stress causes a normal buildup of minerals, mainly calcium, in the bones, and gives them a good strong structure. People who stay in bed for a long time or even those who are sedentary and don't stand very often get weak bones. An extreme loss of minerals causes a hollowing of the bones, a condition called osteoporosis.

The third requirement, lifting a heavy load, can be met by carrying a bag or two of groceries.

If you walk briskly with those groceries in your arms, you will stimulate your cardiovascular system. That's requirement four.

When you're at rest, or moving about in a quiet manner, your motor is effectively idling. The difference between a resting rate of 90 beats a minute and an all-out rate of 180 beats a minute is 90 beats. If you were to take one third of this difference—30 beats—and add it to your idling rate, you'd be moving along at 120 beats a minute when you're in good condition. That's your cruising speed; it's when the organism really purrs. Until you reach good condition, your cruising pulse should be kept near 100 beats a minute.

ACTIVITY CALORIES

Now to the fifth requirement.

What are we talking about when we say you need three hundred calories of physical activity a day in order to prevent physical deterioration? Three hundred above what?

We begin with the basal-metabolic rate. That's the energy required to maintain life: about 1,500 calories a day. You use this up, whether you do anything else or not, just to keep the body going: pumping the heart, breathing, digesting, maintaining body temperature.

Suppose you lead a sedentary life at the lowest level of activity. You get up at a late hour, eat a prepared breakfast, read the newspaper and watch television until lunch. Then you make yourself a sandwich and a glass of milk, eat a piece of fruit and take a nap. In midafternoon the mailman comes, and you read your mail. Then you watch the news until supper. You have a TV dinner in front of your set, then watch your favorite shows until bedtime. You sleep for ten hours.

There are people in their forties who live like

this. They get hypokinetic disease from inactivity. They're about five hundred calories above the basal-metabolic level. But they still aren't doing any fitness-building activities.

Office workers who ride to their jobs, take an elevator to their floor and sit all day use 800 calories a day above their basal-metabolic level for these habits. They're deteriorating, for sure, because their heart rate doesn't increase, they lift no extra weight, they're not on their feet for two hours, they're not moving their joints through a complete range of motion, and they're not using an extra three hundred calories of physical activity. But consider how close they are to good caloric balance: they use 2,300 calories doing next to nothing.

If they were to step up from 2,300 calories to 2,600 calories a day, they would cut the legs out from under creeping obesity—and they would have yet to exercise.

How do you add three hundred activity calories a day without exercising? By a very slight modification in your life style. You simply become a slightly more active person.

Activity calories come from movements that increase your pulse rate above 100 beats a minute. When you've been leading an otherwise sedentary life, any physical movement that increases your pulse twenty beats above resting level steps up your metabolic rate. Walking, lifting, carrying, climbing, sexual activity—any of these will do. Even making ordinary motions more vigorously than you ordinarily make them will burn activity calories.

The housewife who cares daily for a two-bedroom home burns her three hundred activity calories easily; she's walking three to four miles in the process.

The following table will give you an indication of the number of calories per minute you would expend while doing the listed activities.

Activity	Calories Expended per Minute
Walking, 2 mph	2.8
Walking, 3.5 mph	4.8
Bicycling. 5.5 mph	3.2
Bicycling rapidly	6.9
Running. 5.7 mph	12.0
Running, 7.0 mph	14.5
Running. 11.4 mph	21.7
Swimming (crawl), 2.2 mph	26.7
Swimming (breaststroke), 2.2 mph	30.8
Swimming (backstroke), 2.2 mph	33.3
Golf	5.0
Tennis	7.1
Table tennis	5.8
Dancing (fox trot)	5.2

Three hundred calories of exercise means walking three miles a day. This doesn't mean walking three miles continuously; it means walking them at various times during the day. Whether you jog a mile in eight minutes or walk it in twenty minutes, you consume the same number of calories. Shopping is walking; the person who does the shopping in your household could meet his or her daily requirement in the supermarket.

If you want to use your three hundred calories up in one hour or less, you can play tennis, dig in the garden, chop wood and so forth. It's obvious that burning three hundred calories in one bout of exercise is more arduous than most people have the patience or stamina for. The alternative is to work the burning of these calories into the day. If you stretch, stand, lift and move briskly all during the day, you're almost surely burning your three hundred calories.

GYMLESSNASTICS

What follows is a scenario for a typical day in which you will meet all the requirements of minimum maintenance without doing a single exercise.

When you awaken in the morning, enjoy the best yawn you've ever had. This is the moment when you have a natural impulse to stretch. Do it. Think of the way a cat stretches, and take a cue. A cat hasn't been told that it's impolite to yawn and stretch; if we hadn't been put down all our lives, we'd be good yawners and stretchers, too. If you stretch your joints to their extreme length for as long as you feel the urge, you've taken care of your stretching exercises for the day.

When you take a shower or a bath, soap yourself vigorously; instead of wiping yourself dry gently, wipe briskly.

Any kind of polishing activity is good cardiovascular exercise. In addition to its sensuous pleasures, hard toweling of your body can get your heart rate up to 120. Polishing the skin, in addition, takes off the scaly layers. That's all dead tissue out there.

Here's the perfect illustration of a natural moment in the day to help yourself to fitness: you've done nothing artificial, yet you've worked your heart rate up for just the length of time you need. When you go to work or shop, take stairs instead of an elevator. If you take an escalator, walk up the moving stairs. The same for coming down. Walking down is a third as good as walking up, but it's still good exercise. It exercises a different set of muscles in the legs.

An airline pilot I know came to me once complaining that he was getting out of shape. Our conversation led me eventually into a study of muscle weakness among pilots. The program I wrote for the pilots emphasized that they should make use of every opportunity they could to work their bodies. In airports on their way to their craft, they're usually carrying about twenty to thirty pounds of luggage with them. If all they did was carry those bags up the stairs instead of standing on the escalator—or if they would at least walk on the escalator—it could mean the difference between preservation of their condition and deterioration.

The best-conditioned crew member on an airplane isn't the pilot. It's the stewardess. She can ride the escalator if she wants. She's got some hard work ahead of her.

During the day, whether you're in an office or at home, follow these maxims:

- Don't lie down when you can sit.
- Don't sit when you can stand.
- Don't stand when you can move.

Stand up when you take all telephone calls. If you're in an office and you want to talk to someone in the same firm, walk down the hall to see him instead of calling his extension. Stand at his desk when you talk to him.

If there's a typewriter to be carried, or a chair to be moved, welcome the opportunity. Women who are knowledgeable about fitness don't wait for men to help them. They use the opportunity themselves. That single task can be your overload for the day, even if it's only five seconds. An overload —which means, simply, something greater than you're used to doing—should be about half as much as you can lift. There's no need to be precise about it; we don't want you lifting your maximum, and it's not necessary. We know from studies of perception of effort that a person can judge with uncanny accuracy as to his maximum capacities, and portions thereof.

For lunch, pick a restaurant some distance from your office, and walk to it. If you're running errands, park your car a distance from where you're going, or get off the subway or bus one stop early. If you give yourself a four-block walk to get there, the round trip is a mile. Again, it's the distance that counts, not the time you take to get there. If you walk fast or slowly, you get the same calorie burn. If you walk fast, however, you'll get your heart rate up to 120 and meet that requirement for the day. The more briskly you move, the more circulo-respiratory benefit you get.

When you return to work or to your home, treat yourself to some extravagant motions. Yank open the files or the kitchen cabinets. At a conference or a coffee klatch, jump to your feet to make a point, and pace about. Never hold yourself back—move with vigor.

At the end of the day, if you're a working person, walk briskly to your car or train or bus. When you get home, play for a few minutes with your children or your dog. Help with dinner. Set the table. Polish a pan. Fix something that has awaited your attention. Put a section of your library in order. Walk the dog.

In addition to creating opportunities for effort for yourself during the day, you should take advantage of moments of inactivity when you can relax. In traffic, for example, whether you're in your own car or using public transportation, you can utilize the biofeedback principles you used to lower your resting pulse rate. Sink your weight into your seat. Let your feet grow heavy. Let your shoulders fall outward, your face grow slack. A few moments like this during the day will do wonders for your psyche.

I'm often approached by executives who complain that they get spots before their eyes whenever they get into emotional meetings where their budgets or decisions are challenged. I teach them to put their hands on their bellies and make certain the hands rise as they take a breath. Belly breathing is another good way to calm the system.

LOOK FOR FITNESS OPPORTUNITIES

The important principle is not to deprive your body of the things it likes to do. Buy products that haven't taken all the effort away from you. Think what you're depriving yourself of when you invest in an electric garage door opener or a power lawn mower. It's inhuman to unload everything. It kills off the consumer. If you're buying a car, consider getting one with a stick shift. Power steering is nice, but it's expensive, it uses gas and it deprives you of a natural workout that takes not an extra second of time.

When we were figuring out programs to keep the astronauts fit during prolonged space flights, one of the proposals we considered was to beef up all of their activities. Opening up food packages, for example, could be made extremely difficult; if the astronauts didn't exert, they didn't eat. We ultimately decided against that process because the astronauts' situation was so extraordinary. If one of them were injured or fell ill, he would be a burden on the others.

But you don't need to create difficulties for yourself. Exercise can be incorporated into daily life in ways you never suspected, doing the most mundane things. For example, when you wring out your washcloth after you shower or bathe make it an "overload" effort just by squeezing a little harder than you did the last time. An "overload," once again, is an effort just a fraction greater than you're used to exerting. That single action adds new strength to your wrists and arms. To make an exercise out of it, just wring and squeeze the washcloth until the exertion feels moderate; then hold that tension until the exertion feels heavy. That's it. You've exerted about fifty percent of your maximum effort; you've held it long enough to produce a training effect if your muscles are weak, and to maintain strength if your muscles are strong. If you twist the washcloth in the opposite direction, you'll exercise a new set of muscles. Once is enough. For a third exercise, grasp the cloth with both hands, and, holding it near your chest, tug as if pulling it apart until the exertion feels moderate, and hold it until the exertion feels heavy. A fourth exercise: Push the water from the washcloth by pressing your hands together, until the exertion feels moderate. Hold it until the exertion feels heavy.

This whole series takes about a minute. No special equipment, no counting. Your body has told you how much and how long, and you've exercised your hands, wrists, arms, shoulders and chest exactly as much as you need to in order to become fit and remain so.

The idea that you need a special program to stay fit doesn't hold any more water than that washcloth will when you're done with it. The name of the game is frequent and regular activity that contains the five elements—twisting, standing, lifting, a brief burst of motion to get the heart rate up, and sufficient activity to burn 300 calories a day.

If sexual intercourse caused you to exercise all five elements to a sufficient degree, then sexual intercourse would be all you'd need to stay fit. Unfortunately, it seldom gives you all five, and while it increases the heart rate, the increase is emotionally induced, whereas the kind of heart workout you need should come exclusively from physical activity.

If you have a predisposition to be physically active, then you never need worry about doing a formal exercise.

If you meet all five requirements every day, you're comfortably preventing deterioration.

If you met them every other day, you'd be near the edge.

If you don't meet the requirements at all, you'll get below the irreducible minimum.

You have to evaluate where you are. If you had difficulty completing the pulse test, then you're below the minimum level. You're deteriorating. Your first job is to stop your deterioration, and work up to the minimum level.

You don't need an exercise program to bring this condition about. You need only alter your habits by a slight degree. You become slightly more active.

Is this enough? It may be for you. If so, fine. That's the choice you've made. You can operate. You can preserve normal structure and function. You've stopped your decay and erosion.

But if you want to move beyond that plateau, if you want a *reserve* of fitness, so that you don't get tired every day, so that you can meet challenges like changing a tire in the rain, or staying up all night with a sick baby, so that you can enjoy recreational opportunities, such as a long hike, then you'll want to begin your thirty-minutes-a-week program.

X

How to Acquire
a Reserve of Fitness
in Thirty Minutes a Week

To move significantly above the baseline and acquire a reserve of fitness, some planning and regulating of your exercise is in order. You need several different exercises. And each exercise must be performed with an intensity and frequency sufficient to stimulate further conditioning.

That housewife who's flexing, lifting, standing, getting her heart rate up and burning three hundred activity calories every day simply by maintaining her home is certainly not deteriorating. But she's got less than desirable muscle tone and a lack of animal vitality. Reserve, tone and vitality can't be achieved via minimum maintenance; they are the special rewards of three ten-minute bouts of vigorous activity each week.

The objectives of these bouts are twofold: to create good skeletal muscle and to develop circulo-respiratory endurance. There are distinctive exercises for each. Each is important, but of the two the latter is the heart of the pulse-rated conditioning program. Do this if you do nothing else; it's the exercise that will do most to help you live to your fullest and remain fresh and resilient. But do both if you possibly can, because only when circulorespiratory development is located in a comprehensive program of muscle development do you have a program that will serve all your needs.

And it will, no matter how pressed you are. Consider film executive James Aubrey, one-time president of Metro-Goldwyn-Mayer. One day, while we were playing golf together, he told me that his corporate duties had become so great that he could no longer keep fit through his recreational sports. He simply didn't have the time; moreover, he was almost always on the move. He greatly regretted that he had gotten so badly out of shape. When we got back to the clubhouse, I showed him the cabin exercises I had developed in the Navy. Aubrey made me promise to set them down. After refining them, I did. He had such success with them that I passed them on to other executives, and they became the mainstay of our fitness program. The exercises you'll find in this book are the same ones used today by some of the country's major corporate managers.

YOUR MUSCLE DEVELOPMENT PROGRAM

You'll work in three stages of eight weeks each.

In Stage One, you'll develop tissue.

In Stage Two, you'll develop endurance.

In Stage Three, you'll develop strength.

The first priority is to build up muscle bulk. We've got to have tissue to work with. Enlarging the muscle working unit is called muscle "hypertrophying." In weight lifter's terminology, you pack the protein in. The protein is the building block, the part that contracts and makes movement possible. Before you can have movement, you've got to have the engine. Some weight lifters try to speed the process by eating protein supplements and taking protein pills, but the body doesn't store any more than it needs, so the excess is excreted or converted to fat just like any other food. It's exercise that builds the muscles.

Once you have mass, you'll infuse it with blood capillaries, and make chemical changes in the muscle that will provide endurance. You'll then be able to contract the muscle many times when you run, ski, play tennis or work.

Now you have the material you need, the circulation and the chemistry, The third step is to train the nervous system and make further modifications in the chemistry of the muscle, in order to develop strength.

It's important to understand the difference between muscular strength and muscular endurance.

Muscle strength is the ability to lift heavy loads for short periods. Muscle endurance is the ability to sustain work for a long period of time. The two are entirely distinct. You can be terrifically strong and have very little endurance. If we took a prizefighter who had trained for pure strength and put him in the ring with one who had trained for pure endurance, the latter would have to stay out of the former's way for the first couple of rounds, but thereafter would be able to carry the fight. The fighter who trained for pure strength would have to land his knockout blow in the first or second round. After that, he'd be finished. Fighters today don't want big arms, because they would have a lot of weight to support while keeping their arms out. Rather, they want big shoulders that help them send their arms forcefully against an opponent. When you see a fighter with big arms, you can be sure his guard will have fallen by the fourth or fifth round. Fighters train with this in mind. Force equals mass times acceleration. If you have a great mass and you can't move it very fast, you don't have much force. But a slender piece of straw can pierce a telephone pole when driven with great velocity by the wind.

The exercises used to build bulk are completely different from those used to build power or endurance. You shouldn't work for all three at once. You may use the same exercise, but you do it in a totally different way. In Stage One, muscle development, you aren't ready to do the exercise you'll do in Stage Three for strength; you simply won't have enough muscle. You couldn't begin your program with the endurance training of Stage Two and expect to develop bulk. Not only would you develop a meager amount of new tissue, you wouldn't develop much endurance. It would be like building a house without a foundation. By Stage Three, you'll be in such good shape, with so much new tissue conditioned for endurance, that you can begin a strength program with ease.

Bulk alone will not give you strength. You can

build mass without getting strong. You can get strong without building mass. If you want mass, you can use a pumping rhythm fifteen to twenty times at seventy percent of your capacity. But it doesn't give you much strength. If you want strength, you exert your maximum one to five times. But it doesn't give you much bulk.

This muscle-building portion of your thirty-minutes-a-week program takes only four minutes a day, three days a week, for the first sixteen weeks, and two minutes a day, three days a week, for the last eight weeks. After twenty-four weeks, you'll have a sound skeletal muscle system with well-supplied tissues. You'll be strong. You'll have endurance. Your total investment of time: exactly four hours.

WHEN?

Whenever. The hour doesn't matter. Any time that's convenient is okay. You can exercise when you awaken, before or after a meal. If you're on a weight-loss program, it might be a good idea to exercise before lunch in order to kill your appetite. If, after exercising, you don't feel like eating, skip it.

Some people might want to exercise before they go to bed as a means of working off the tensions of the day. That's the time I like to exercise the most. I find that a relaxing bath after exercise prepares me nicely for bed. I feel my muscle tone. I feel languorously alive.

The only recommendation as to schedule is that you work out on alternate days—Monday, Wednesday and Friday, or Tuesday, Thursday and Saturday. Sunday is makeup day.

One advantage of exercising first thing in the morning or before retiring is that you can do it at home, in your underwear. Once again, remember the injunction against sweat suits. You want to exercise your muscle system, not your temperature-regulating system. You want to be able to control your effort; once you're overheated, you're out of control. So dress lightly. For men, underwear shorts are perfect. Women can wear panties and bra. A bra is particularly important for women with heavy breasts.

REMINDERS

Before we get under way, let's restate our principles.

At the outset, anything you do will benefit you. Your first week of exercise—just thirty minutes— could put you as much as twenty percent along the road to your final goal, if you're starting from a low point of fitness. At this low level, it's easy to overdo. Remember, there's no hurry. Be sure to monitor your pulse, and remain within the limits you've set for yourself. At the earliest stages, any pulse rate above your base rate means progress.

We used to think it was the last repetition of an

exercise that gave you the most benefit. Today we know it's the initial effort that makes the best contribution to your fitness. The second effort gives you some additional benefit, the third a little less additional benefit, and so on. The farther you go, the less effect each one has. In the case of a champion, these little infinite improvements make the difference between winning and losing in a close race. But in our case these extensions of effort aren't necessary. The athlete must continue his activity even though he feels fatigue and pain, in order to get these infinite improvements. At the fitness level, fatigue and pain are unessential.

When you're exercising for several minutes, as in circulo-respiratory training, you get infinitely more out of the first minute of exercise than you do out of the last. A little is very good—and more is that much better. It would be great if you could complete the recommended number of minutes, but it's no big deal if you don't. You may stop whenever you want. Hopefully, you'll be able to go a little further the next time.

Target times aren't part of your program.

You're not competing against anyone—least of all yourself.

You're in charge of your program. By taking your pulse, you'll know exactly what effect you're producing.

As you proceed , you'll be in better shape, so the same effort will have less effect on you. You'll be able to feel it when you're not getting a sufficient workout. As soon as that happens, increase your effort.

You'll know immediately that you're more fit. You'll feel that a load has been lifted. You'll have better tone, be more relaxed.

After you've exercised for a few weeks, your resting heart rate will drop as much as ten beats a minute.

Remember, you'll probably gain a little weight—perhaps a pound or two—at the outset of your program. This is an event to celebrate, not bemoan. It demonstrates that your body is beginning to change in a manner that will endure. Muscle tissue weighs more than fatty tissue. As muscle replaces fat, the scale will reflect it. What's more important than your scale is what you see in the mirror.

Exercise should be enjoyable. You should approach it with the conviction that you're going to have some fun. If you don't keep your back straight or your hands and elbows in just the right position, who cares? There's no drill sergeant to scold you. The important thing is to involve the muscles and their supporting systems in a stimulating way.

Your program suggests that you perform a few repetitions of an exercise, or keep your pulse rate up near a certain level for a few minutes. These aren't standards of excellence we're asking you to achieve. They have nothing to do with the time or distance or number of points you have to score. They stem solely from the knowledge of what it takes to get you into shape.

Above all, let your body tell you what your exercise should be. It will tell you if you haven't had enough. It will tell you when you've had too much.

You should never feel sore or tired after your exercise. You should feel good.

PRECAUTIONS

We'll keep them to a minimum, but there are a few precautions to observe in exercising that are important for your health. We've mentioned them before, but let's get them all in one place.

Never hold your breath and strain. Many weight lifters' gyms teach their members to hold their breath when they're lifting a weight. The assumption is that the air will somehow support the chest. This is just another one of those myths. The simple rule of breathing in all exercise is to always keep the glottis open. The glottis is a valve in your throat; you can close it voluntarily and stop the process of exhalation. When you do that and at the same time continue to try to exhale, your diaphragm and rib cage contract to increase the pressure inside the thorax, or chest. The pressure buildup within the chest becomes greater than the pressure in the veins returning blood to the heart. This clamps off the flow and deprives the heart of blood. The heart soon pumps itself empty. The result is a fall in pressure. The brain is the first organ to sense this fall in pressure. Result: fainting or blackout. No good weight lifter will close his glottis as he strains. He will either suck or whistle air. You should do the same when exercising.

A related precaution, and a vital one, ought to be mentioned here. Many people either die or come close to death on the toilet at night due to heart attacks or strokes. The typical episode is when a person awakens with a pain in his stomach or chest, which he attributes to gas. He figures he should go to the bathroom. Immediately on sitting, he feels better. But then he finds he can neither defecate nor pass gas. So he strains at the stool, closing his glottis in an attempt to increase the intra-abdominal pressure and thereby force an excretion. The coronaries depend on the heart for blood. As soon as they empty out, bam. The general rule of life is: Never close your glottis.

Keep your water level high. Remember, if you're going to work out first thing in the morning, drink a glass of water first. During your workout, don't even wait until you're thirsty to have some water. On an especially warm, dry day you should have a glass of water every half hour at least.

Take a sufficient warmup. You don't want to embarrass your heart. If you start from a condition of rest and run full tilt up a hill, that might prove embarrassing. The heart will be forced to work too hard before the circulation in the coronary system has had a chance to adjust and supply sufficient blood. This causes a condition called myocardial ischemia—i.e., insufficient circulation, with the heart muscle deprived of oxygen. In a healthy person this may not be dangerous, but it could trigger a heart attack in someone who isn't fit.

Warming up consists of increasing your activity gradually from very light (100 pulse) to moderate intensity (120 pulse). Doing this over a period of one minute is just about as good as taking six or twelve minutes. A prolonged warmup is a way to avoid getting into your exercise; it wastes time and adds nothing to your workout. After your minute of warmup there is no need to rest, or no need to hurry into exercise. Just go ahead at your own pace.

The best warmup you can take is to rehearse slowly what you're going to do more actively later on. But once again, don't overdo it. Moderation is the order. It's good to move your joints to a full range of motion in order to prevent tying up. But violent and forceful bending and stretching can cause the opposite effect; you induce a reactive contraction of the muscle, which gets you tied up even worse than you might have been had you not warmed up at all. Overstretched ligaments can weaken joints, such as ankles and knees, and invite injuries.

My office at UCLA is in the men's gym, across the street from the athletic field. At the opposite end of the field is Drake Stadium, where the university championship track and field team works out. One day I happened to look over toward the stadium and saw four men warming up before practice. They were doing typical exercises, such as the hurdler's stretch, in which you put one heel on top of the hurdle and dive toward your ankle, or sit on the ground in a straddle position, one leg forward, the other bent to the side, and trunk-twist with your arms extended. I walked over and said, "Do you have fifteen minutes? I'd like you to come to the lab. I want to check something." When we got to the Human Performance Laboratory, I measured the flexibility of their hips and trunks. "Now do those exercises again that you were doing on the field," I asked. They did. I measured them once again. All of them had lost flexibility. Their tissues were becoming tight by reactive contraction —just the opposite effect from the increased range of motion they wanted.

The best warmup for a golf match is a golf swing—but not with more than one club, and not with a weighted club. When I see baseball players swinging several bats, or one bat with a ringed weight on it, I wince. In both cases, you get the feeling of extra power, but all you've done is confuse your kinesthetic sense. Your performance will deteriorate. It's all right to use weighted devices for strengthening your arms. But they should be used in practice, never in a warmup. If you do use them as a warmup, then be sure you use the implement you're actually going to use in the sport half a dozen times at least before you actually perform. In that way, you'll erase this kinesthetic ghost.

In your fitness program, you'll be doing four simple stretching exercises. They're ample preparation for your workout.

One supplementary caution: If you jog, don't jog downhill. Not long ago, a group of members at my country club formed a jogging group. Before long they had to stop exercising entirely, because their knees were giving out. They had difficulty walking and climbing stairs. They came to me for an explanation. I told them that jogging or running downhill puts a terrific strain on the knees. The rule: Run up, walk down.

Walk around, or sit down, after exercising. The body doesn't like to be quiet after exercise. It's restless. It wants to move. Gravity tries constantly to force your body fluids into your lower extremities. If that happens, blood drains from the brain, and you faint. You're particularly vulnerable when you exercise. Then the vessels throughout your body open wide to increase circulation to the working muscles. As long as you're working, the skeletal muscles act as pumps to keep the blood flowing back to the heart. If you stop exercising suddenly and stand quietly, then you're relying on the heart muscle alone to pump the blood—and that's not enough. The vessels remain in an open state, they still need blood. The increase in demand means a decrease in supply to some part of the body. Gravity makes the choice. You can actually measure the swelling in the ankles of someone who stands quietly after vigorous exercise.

One afternoon while we were preparing this book, my collaborator, Leonard Gross, took a tennis lesson from his professional, "Lefty" Willner. Midway through the lesson, Lefty called Leonard to the net to give him some instruction.

"Do you mind if we sit down?" Leonard said.

"Are you feeling bad?" Lefty asked.

"No," Leonard said. He then explained the above phenomenon.

"I'll be damned," Lefty said. "I've had people faint on me at the net. I'll be talking to them, and they'll just drop. I could never figure out why."

Easy does it. Recently my neighbor Hal Hoag, a gentleman of fifty-seven years, had a valve installed in his heart. He was in bed for nearly two months following surgery. During bed rest there's a loss of muscle tissue and circulatory tissue, which we call arterioles and capillaries. To the extent that anyone is inactive, this loss occurs as well, so what happened to Hal has important bearing on fitness programs.

Hal was anxious to get back to his previous level of activity. He has a tendency to push himself as far as he can as fast as he can. He began his recuperation by walking. His legs recovered their girth in about a month. But they also ached. The reason they did is that muscle tissue recovers about six times faster than circulatory tissue. Hal was soon strong enough to walk appreciable distances and up the stairs, but his circulatory system was incapable of supplying the working muscles with the fuels they needed. Nor could the circulatory system wash away the lactic acids, the waste products of muscular activity. When lactic acid accumulates in the tissue, the tissues swell. This swelling irritates the sensory nerves, causing first a burning sensation and then pain.

What happened to Hal can happen to the rest of us if we exercise too fast. You have to plan your exercise program in accordance with the rate of development of different physiological systems. You'll quickly develop more strength than you can comfortably use. If you tax your endurance, you'll get stiff. Getting stiff is simply the accumulation of lactic acid or other metabolites in the working tissues. It is *not* an indication that you're getting strong, as most gym instructors will tell you. There's no need to get stiff. You won't if you ease into increased activity.

OVERLOAD

We've all heard about the legendary Milo of Crotona who lifted a baby ox from the day that the beast was born. Each day the ox got bigger. Each day the man grew stronger. Finally the ox was full grown, and the man was still able to lift him.

The story is apocryphal, but the principle it illustrates is real.

Overload is the foundation of your fitness program, and the main ingredient of training. It is based on the biological law of adaptation. In the study of bones, the first thing we learn is Wolf's Law: structure follows function. This means that the construction of a bone conforms not only to the degree of use but to the manner of use as well. By reading the internal architecture of a bone, you can tell the past history of that bone. The more a bone is used, the thicker and heavier it gets. The more twisting and turning to which the bone is subject, the more its internal structure organizes to resist that kind of stress.

Today we're finding that muscle follows essentially the same law. This includes the heart muscle. Sur-

geons have learned that if you remove a portion
of a muscle, or transplant a muscle to an unusual
position, the muscle will restructure itself to conform with the demands made on it. In four words:
Use makes the organ.

Body tissues and their capabilities are highly
adaptable. Body functions—strength, the ability to
contract, the ability to support a load—deteriorate
with disuse. If you don't use bones, they dissolve.
The minerals leach out of the bones. They become
more porous, lightweight and fragile—the condition
called osteoporosis.

It's when the reverse situation applies that a
training effect occurs.

No matter how poor one's physical condition
has become, and no matter what his age, his physical condition can be improved by applying loads
in gradually increased amounts.

Your program works every muscle you need to
use, plus your cardiovascular system. But it's the
manner in which your program puts muscles and
systems to use that is crucial.

Each workout has an achievement objective that
hasn't been previously achieved. *You don't have
a program if you're only doing a number of exercises the same number of times.* It becomes a program only when you incorporate the principle of
progressive overload.

You'll start just above the level of your ordinary
activity. If the heaviest object you're used to lifting
weighs ten pounds, then your training program starts
at eleven pounds. If your heart rate never exceeds

90, then your training program starts at 100. If you never walked more than three blocks, your program starts with four blocks. You should always feel you're a great success every time you do a fraction more today than you did yesterday.

WAYS TO OVERLOAD

If you're fairly active, and then suddenly stop being active for several days, you'll gradually lose your fitness to be active. Each day you'll be less fit than the day before. Even within any twenty-four-hour period, there is a slight but measurable reduction in fitness whether you've been active or not. So, in effect, if you do the same activity today that you did yesterday, it is really an "overload," because by today you have become slightly de-adapted to the activity you did yesterday. This "overload" today stimulates a readaptation—which will fade slightly by tomorrow.

A uniform activity level is okay for maintenance, but if you want to become fit at a higher level of activity than you are used to, you will have to assume a greater "overload."

There are many ways to "overload." The most risky way is to increase the *intensity* of the effort: to lift a heavier load, or to move faster, or to move against heavier resistance. A safer way is to increase the *duration* of the effort: to carry the load a little farther, to hang on a little longer. The safest way is to increase the *frequency* of the effort: do it one more time a week. Those who train by lifting weights do each exercise a number of times, which they call a "set." They progressively overload by either increasing the number of lifts each set, or by increasing the number of sets. They adjust the weights so that the desired frequency in terms of lifts, or sets, can be completed during each session.

To elevate your exercise heart rate to a new stage, you can move a little faster. For the next higher stage you can add a little resistance: heavier shoes while running in place, or choosing a little steeper incline for your brisk walk. If the grade is more than you expected and your heart rate is rising too much, just slow your pace a bit or rest occasionally. Make a wide variety of adjustments in the way you exercise, but keep to your desired exercise heart rate.

Another way to achieve progressive overload is to gradually increase the effort during your rest period. In other words, don't wait until the heart rate gets to the resting level before you start the next bout of activity. Maintain a more constant level of stimulus. Instead of sitting, walk around, flex, be active in any way you like.

Yet another way to achieve progressive overload is to gradually shorten the rest periods until you have virtually eliminated them.

It's you who continually adjust the intensity of your exercises. To develop muscles, start at fifteen contractions. Each bout you try to work up to twenty. When you've succeeded, make the exercise ever so slightly more difficult, and drop back to fifteen.

Instead of laying out a program of progressive exercise on the basis of the number of times you do an exercise, we do it on the basis of your body's reaction to the work. We let a very accurate mechanism inside you, your perception of the intensity of exercise, be your guide.

You can use that marvelous computer, your pulse, as your guide to the speed of movement. If you feel any discomfort whatever—breathlessness, pain, cramping, whatever—stop the exercise for the day. But if all is well, as your condition improves you'll have to step faster is order to keep your heart rate at the prescribed level. This is part of the automatic feedback in the system.

YOUR TRAINING PULSE RATE

The accompanying chart will locate your Training Pulse Rate for each eight-week period if you are just starting a fitness program. If you're already training at a higher pulse rate, there is no need to fall back to a lower rate.

The Training Pulse Rate is figured by multiplying the difference between 220 and your age by sixty percent the first period, seventy percent the second, and eighty percent the third and thereafter.

If you're forty years old, for example, the remainder from 220 is 180. Multiplied by .60, that's 108. We round it off to 110.

Age	TPR-1	TPR-2	TPR-3	TPR-4
Under 30	120	140	150	150–160
30–44	110	130	140	140–150
45–60	100	120	130	130–140
Over 60	100	110	120	120–130

TPR = Training Pulse Rate.

TPR-1 = TPR for the first 8 weeks—about 60% maximum PR (220 minus your age, × .60).

TPR-2 = TPR for the second 8 weeks—about 70% maximum PR.

TPR-3 = TPR for the third 8 weeks—about 80% maximum PR.

TPR-4 = TPR to maintain total fitness.

I don't want you to become a compulsive pulse counter. Use your pulse as a checkpoint to gauge the accuracy of your perception of exertion, so that you can find the intensity which is just right for you. Usually a feeling of "mild" or "moderate" exertion, one which is neither light nor heavy, during continuous effort is matched by a pulse rate of about 120 per minute. After you have once established your perception of exertion level, you need only to check it against your pulse once in a while. As your condition improves you'll notice that you're doing more work (walking faster, pedaling harder) to produce the same "moderate" level—and your pulse stays about the same, 120 per minute. If your condition deteriorates due to a layoff or slight illness, the same exertion iwll produce less work. You'll walk slower or cycle less hard to reach the "moderate" level.

Here's a good example of your inner computer at work. When Jim Youngblood, the executive administrator of NASA, learned about our program with the astronauts, he decided to try a portion of it himself. His office was on the fifth floor of the administration building of the Johnson Space Center in Houston. His idea was to jog all five flights. We told him to go ahead, but not to let his pulse get over 120. In the first weeks, he had to stop frequently before reaching the fifth floor. Within three months, he had to practically run up the stairs to work his pulse up to 120.

Without incorporating pulse rate, the most sophisticated exercise programs won't work. Standardized regimens promise that if you adhere to a certain schedule, your performance will increase to a certain level without fail. True enough. You'll get a certain performance. But what's the performance doing to you? It may be doing almost nothing. Or it may be killing you. Electronic programs are faulty for the same reason. In these, the load is set up so that each time you can challenge yourself to do a little more. The two embodying ideas are motivation and progressive overload. But if you don't know your physiological parameters and where such exercise puts you within them, you could be hurting yourself—or spinning your wheels. There's just no way to tell, unless you take your pulse.

XI

Three Short Steps to Fitness

What follows applies equally to men and women. The exercises are the same because the requirements are the same. Women need good muscles every bit as much as men do. To obtain good muscles, they must first develop a certain quantity of tissue. Then they must develop two muscle qualities, endurance and strength. Their work or sport requires both. Finally, the circulo-respiratory endurance of a woman is no less vital to her health and fitness than is that of a man.

As a general rule, men like to get their work done in bursts. Women don't care to push that much. Our program combines both time dimensions. Each session is compact; it asks you to concentrate your effort into one brief time span. There's no way around that requirement, because you need to raise your heart rate to be fit, and only compact action does that. But the fitness program itself spreads out over twenty-four weeks, and continues throughout your lifetime.

Each of you will start these exercises according

to your readiness for them. Each of you will make the exercises a little bit more difficult according to your individual capacity to extend. The degree of difficulty doesn't matter, so long as it's a slight overload for *you*. Don't compare what you're doing with what anyone else is doing.

STEP ONE

During the first eight weeks your ten-minute exercise session will be divided up into three parts:

1. One minute of limbering.
2. Four minutes of muscle building.
3. Five minutes of any continuous activity that raises your heart rate to the desired level.

Limbering

The object of these four limbering exercises is to increase your range of motion so that you can move more easily. There is no drill. Use whatever rhythm pleases you. Don't count; there's no need. Just spend about fifteen seconds on each exercise.

1. Reach up as high as you can toward the ceiling with one arm. Your hand should be directly over your head. It's a prolonged reach we're after. Feel the stretch all the way to your ankle, all the way along your side. When you feel all stretched out,

drop your arm, and repeat the exercise with your other arm. Be a cat; stretch to your outer limit.

2. Arms extended sideward, twist your trunk in either direction as far as you can turn. Then twist in the opposite direction. In the military, this

LIMBERING

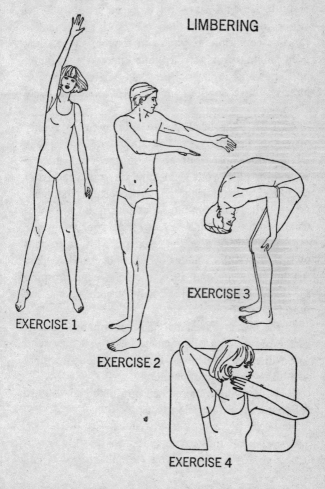

EXERCISE 1

EXERCISE 2

EXERCISE 3

EXERCISE 4

exercise is performed with a snap. These are non-military proceedings. No snaps, please.

3. Lean over, grasp yourself behind the knees with your hands, and pull your shoulders gently toward your knees. Don't use force. Don't use momentum. Just an easy stretch. Some people will get closer to their knees than others. It's all relative to your condition. If you're in terrible shape, then even gaining proximity to your knees is a triumph, and you've done yourself a world of good. If you're already fairly supple, you should soon get fairly close.

4. Turn your head to the side, with your chin over the top of your left shoulder. Place your left hand against your chin, on the right side of your face. Place your right hand on your head from behind. Left and right hands now turn the head just a little farther than it can turn on its own. Gently, please. Don't try to jerk your head, or snap it. Now reverse the process, with your chin over your right shoulder, your right hand against the left side of your face, the left hand grasping the head from behind. Slowly stretch your neck muscles.

In the first few sessions, one performance of each of the movements is sufficient. Later you may wish to do them twice or even three times. But do them in a leisurely, languid manner.

Now that you are stretched and limbered you are ready to develop muscle tissue.

Muscle Buildup

During the next four minutes you're going to concentrate on developing muscle fibers by pumping motions of your muscles, against resistance. As you continue to exercise, it will be easier for you to overcome the same resistance. So you should gradually increase the resistance.

You'll do two exercises, alternating them for a full four minutes. The first will expand the muscles of your shoulders, chest and arms. The second will expand the muscles of your abdomen and back. Don't worry about your legs, they'll get all the exercise they need at the end of this session.

1. Expansion Pushaways

Stand a little beyond arm's reach from a wall. Put your hands against the wall at the height of your shoulders. Lean forward until your chest comes near the wall. Then push away until you're back in the starting position. If that's too hard, step in closer. Do the exercise about fifteen or twenty times, or until the exertion begins to feel heavy. This is one *set*.

If the exercise was a workout for you at a set of fifteen pushaways or less, keep at it each session.

When you can do a set of twenty or more with ease, move to a position with the feet farther away from the wall.

In successive workouts you'll be able to do more

repetitions. Just keep backing away from the wall until you find the position that gives a moderate effort. If you can do a set of more than twenty pushaways before the exertion begins to feel heavy, shift to a new position next time.

Some people will find at the outset that the pushaway from the wall is too easy. In that event, try a kitchen counter, or a bathroom sink, or a chest of drawers—anything that lowers the height of your hands below the height of your shoulders. If you can do only fifteen pushaways before the exertion becomes heavy, you've found your starting place. We want an exercise that begins to feel difficult after fifteen executions. At each session, you'll be adding more repetitions as your condition improves. When you can do a set of more than twenty with only a mild effort, increase the difficulty of the pushaway exercise.

PUSHAWAY
(height of hands below shoulders position)

From the counter or sink or chest of drawers, move next to a table, and repeat the same routine.

From the table, move to a chair or a bench.

From the chair or bench, move to the floor. Put your knees on the floor. When you're able to do a set of twenty pushaways, try them with your knees off the floor. Pushaways in this floor position are commonly called "pushups."

For the person who is in fairly good shape to begin with, twenty pushaways in the above positions may soon become too easy, He can increase the resistance by reversing the process that made it simpler. Instead of having his hands higher than his feet, he moves his feet higher than his hands. They are placed first on a low bench, then on a chair, then on a table, etc., until the extreme case, when the feet are over the head. None of us will likely get there; none of us needs to; but it's a good illustration of the many ways in which the difficulty of our pushaway exercise can be increased.

2. Expansion Sitbacks

This exercise will restore the muscles of your abdominal wall.

The abdominal muscles are the hardest ones to involve in beneficial exercise. They're supportive muscles, not meant to flex isotonically—i.e., with movement. They function isometrically, holding without moving, and that's the way they should be exercised.

Whenever you do an ordinary isotonic "situp," there's a tendency to call on two larger hip flexor muscles, the psoas and the iliacus, to do most of the

work, and to leave the abdominal muscles out of
it. Some time ago I started searching for an exercise that would overcome this problem and really
give the abdominals a workout. Using electromyo-
graphic studies of the muscles during various movements, I found a simple solution: to reverse the
process. If you started with your chest at your
knees and went backward, instead of rising from
the floor to your knees, the abdominals would act
in their normal manner, as supporting muscles,
while the body was being lowered.

In the traditional situp, it's almost impossible
for the abdominal muscles to bring the shoulders
up without strongly involving the psoas and iliacus
muscles.

On the way back, the tendency is to relax the
abdominal muscles and collapse. As a consequence,
the muscles getting the best workout are those that
don't profit from it—the hip flexors. The exercise
tends to foreshorten them; they're already too short
as is.

In the *sitback,* it's almost impossible to move
backward without involving the abdominal muscles. You don't need an electromyograph to check
those; you can do it yourself just by touching
the abdominal muscles with your fingers. You'll feel
them harden as they come into action, and soften
as they relax.

The sitback has a psychological as well as physiological advantage over the situp. For the person
who's out of condition, the situp can be all but
impossible. There's no way to reduce the difficulty
beyond a certain minimum. You've got to get off

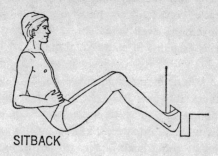

SITBACK

the floor. The sitback permits every degree of difficulty.

We're not interested in how far back you go. We're interested in exercising you to your own personal degree of effort. We define this degree as a moderate effort, meaning it's neither easy nor difficult. But you're the one who gauges that effort in terms of your own resources. When you've gone back to a point where the return will be moderately difficult, that's a good workout for you.

In whatever position you do the expansion sitback, remember to oppose the tendency to hold your breath. Keep breathing.

Sit on the floor, feet hooked under a piece of furniture. Fully bend your knees. Work your chest up against your knees, or as closely as it will come. Place your hands on your abdomen so that you can feel the muscle action. If you're not trained to exercise, you may not be able to bring your abdominal muscle voluntarily into action. A good way to teach your muscles to respond is by a biofeedback technique. Probe the abdominal muscles with your fingers while trying to harden them, and feel the hardness with your fingers as the muscles contract. The muscle signals its response to the exercise. Even when you're trained, probing with your fingers will cause your muscle to harden even more.

Once you're in position, move back away from your knees until you feel your abdominal musculature coming into play to a moderate degree. To find this moderate degree, it's necessary to explore. Start out by going back just a few inches, and then return. If that was easy, go back a few more inches, and return. Keep it up until you've found the spot where you're getting a mild workout. Once again, the body is a good estimator of what it can do. It may be that you'll go back too far on one occasion to a point where you can't make it back to the starting position. If that happens, just let yourself collapse to the floor, use your arms to get yourself into the starting position again, and resume the exercise. Now your position for moderate exertion has been extremely well defined.

As your condition improves, your point of moderate effort will drop farther and farther backward. Eventually, your shoulder blades will lightly brush the floor.

Start with a degree of effort that enables you to *hold the position for fifteen to twenty seconds*. The last few seconds the belly muscles will begin to quiver. Work up to a full twenty-second sitback before quivering commences, then try a deeper sitback. When your back is brushing the floor, and you can hold the sitback for twenty seconds or more, you can proceed to "load up" the exercise by moving your arms. You've been holding them in front of you, with your hands on your stomach. Now fold them on your chest in order to increase the resistance. That little change will take you back to fifteen seconds per set; you may even need to make your sitback more shallow for a few days.

The next position is arms folded and resting on your chest. When that has been mastered, move your hands behind your head. Finally, move your arms over your head. Caution: Don't swing your arms. They're elevated for added weight, and should not be used for momentum.

You don't get points for advancing in difficulty. You're doing it only to make personal adjustments. You're getting just as much value out of the first position, relative to your condition at the time, as you are from the last position at the time you employ it.

Important: After one set each of the muscle buildup exercises, check your pulse to be sure it isn't over your limit, sixty percent of your maximum level. If it is, rest. After a few weeks your pulse rate will be coming down because the other work you're doing will be strengthening your circulorespiratory system. There's absolutely no need to exceed the goal you've established for your first eight-week period. Your internal computer, your pulse, will be making the achievement of that goal increasingly more difficult as you proceed.

Now repeat the sets of muscle buildup exercises in the same order and again monitor your pulse. You may not be able to hold the sitback position for as long the second time around. That's par for the course. Maintain the same exercise until you can. Then increase the duration of the effort on the first set.

The double sets usually take about four minutes. The remaining five minutes of your ten-minute program are devoted to your heart-rated circulo-respiratory conditioning.

Circulo-respiratory Endurance "Lope"

You can choose any steady, easy activity you want that will raise your heart rate to your proper level for five minutes during this phase.

The loping activity should be a rhythmic, continuous exercise. The reason I recommend leg action over arm action at the outset is that arm action tends to elevate blood pressure more than leg action. Armwork, such as rowing, is best postponed until the circulatory system is better adjusted to exercise.

The most obvious steady, easy endurance exercise is running in place. It's also the most boring. The second most obvious exercise is jogging. For most people it's the second most boring. Do either if you wish. Or try the Fitness Hop.

The generation that grew up in the sixties liberated the dance form until it became an expression of feeling. I'd be honored to do as much for exercise. Surely you've danced at some point in your life—the Charleston, the Twist, the Shimmy. All I'd like you to do now is dance once more, in any way you like, for five minutes. The only requirement is that your movements be energetic

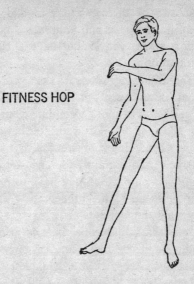

FITNESS HOP

enough to get your pulse rate up to your moderate level by the end of the second minute, and to maintain that level for another three minutes.

If the spirit moves you, you might want to try incorporating the Fitness Hop into your movements. Hop twice on the left foot, then twice on the right foot, then twice on both feet. Repeat. If there's a radio or record player handy, tune in and turn on. Otherwise, you can hum or whistle or just think of a tune. The rhythm of "Tea for Two" is particularly effective for the Fitness Hop. If you're meditating, get your mantra going.

Don't forget: Move around when you take your pulse. Never come to a complete standstill. The same applies to the end of your workout.

That's your program for this phase. It should

take you two or three sessions to find your patterns, positions, speed and endurance. By the end of the first week, you should have a comfortable ten-minute routine.

For the following seven weeks, your only requirement is to keep intensifying your activity. Stretch farther. Put more vigor into your workout. Change the position of your pushaways. Shift your arms when doing your sitbacks.

On your cardiovascular endurance lope, that intensification is automatic. You have to do more to get your pulse up to the proper beat. That's your own internal computer at work.

A reminder: Your proper beat is calculated by subtracting your age from 220, then multiplying the remainder by sixty percent. Example: 220 minus 40 = 180; 180 × .60 = 108. Call it 110. That's your starting Training Pulse Rate. Don't fall back if you're trained at a higher level.

STEP TWO

Now you've got some muscles, not to look bulky—you won't—but to hold your frame erect, give you some confidence in yourself and move you where you want to go. Our next job is to give those muscles a capacity for *endurance,* so that any sudden situation requiring extra effort won't throw you off schedule for a week.

We're also going to move up a notch in our circulo-respiratory conditioning. Again, the aim is endurance.

Muscle Endurance

We no longer have to worry about expansion—the building of muscle tissue. By now, you've got all the bulk you need. Nor do we need to worry about range of motion. If you're doing enough stretching in your minimum-maintenance program, that's enough. However, you may want to do the limbering routines as a warmup before your workouts in this phase.

The second eight weeks require a new series of training methods to achieve the new objectives. We'll utilize the first four minutes for muscle endurance training, the last six for circulo-respiratory endurance training. Now that we have an improved heart and circulation, we're going to start pushing the new capillaries into skeletal muscles. This will induce the chemical and structural changes necessary to give the muscle cells the endurance they need for prolonged activities such as tennis, skiing, carpentry, gardening and so on.

We're also going to take up *interval training,* which helps us get the heart rate up to higher levels without fatigue. But first, let's work on the muscles.

1. Endurance Pushaways

Your first exercise is to do twice as many pushaways as you were doing in Step One, and feel that the exertion is moderate at the end; not light, not heavy. In order to do that many without a heavy effort, you'll have to lighten the resistance considerably from what it was at the end of that first eight weeks, when you were exercising for muscle bulk. It may be that you had worked your way from the wall through all the stages to the floor. Nonetheless, it would be a good idea to go back to the wall the first time you try to do about forty pushaways. If that's too easy, try the next hardest level the next time you exercise.

The objective is to do twice as many, *and do them fast*.

You'll adjust the intensity by moving your feet away from the wall. Start at just beyond arm's length. Once again, if that's too hard, step in closer. The important thing is to be able to do about forty pushaways. If you can easily do more than fifty, you're standing too close. Once you've found the position that enables you to just barely get forty without the exercise becoming heavy, maintain that position until you can get a moderate exertion at about fifty. Then move to the next position. As you step away from the wall, you automatically increase the load.

Pushaways from the wall can be very easy if you stand next to the wall, but if you get back far enough you'll find them an interesting challenge.

Doing forty to fifty pushaways isn't a rigid rule. It's just an order of magnitude. In order to gain endurance, you have to do relatively lighter work rapidly for a greater number of times. If you quit before twenty, you're not doing an endurance exercise. If you get thirty-five and have to stop, or if you get sixty without feeling tired, fine, that's your workout for the day. Make adjustments the next time you exercise. Stand closer or farther away; go faster or slower.

2. Endurance Sitbacks

Assume the same position you did for the regular sitback—on the floor, knees bent, feet hooked under or around a piece of furniture.

Now lean back just a little, about a third of the way to the floor. *Hold that position for ten or fifteen seconds.* Next, move back a notch, so that you're approximately halfway between your starting position and the floor. *Again, hold for ten to fifteen seconds.* Finally, move back to the three-quarter position, *and try to hold that for ten to fifteen seconds.*

While you're leaning backward, probe the abdominal muscles in all areas, low and high, with your hands. This helps to keep the muscles hardened.

When the exertion starts to become heavy, your belly will begin to quiver. That's your signal to straighten up or relax backward onto the floor.

It may take you a few days to establish just how far back you should go. If you're back too far, you'll start to quiver before thirty seconds. If you're too far forward, you won't quiver until after forty seconds.

As soon as you've finished the sitback, do another set of endurance pushaways.

When you've finished the second set of endurance pushaways, do another set of endurance sitbacks.

Two sets each of two exercises should take you four minutes. If you find that you can't do the four sets in four minutes, then do as many as you can. Don't hurry yourself, but try to develop to a point where you can do two sets of each exercise. If you can get only thirty pushaways on the second set, fine. If you can hold the sitback for only twenty seconds the second time, also fine. You'll soon get to a point where you can easily do four complete sets in four minutes.

Reminder: Check your heart rate every two minutes. Keep it within prescribed limits. Your upper limit is now seventy percent of 220 minus your age. Example: 220 minus 40 = 180; 180 × .70 = 126. The nearest interval of ten is 130. You can go to 130 beats a minute, or thirteen beats in six seconds. No higher, please—unless you've been exercising at a more advanced TPR.

Circulo-respiratory Endurance Intervals

Now, interval training.

It consists of six minutes of exertion in which sallies of intensive exercise are alternated with intervals of active rest. The conventional method is to run for a number of seconds, say thirty, then slow to a walk for about thirty seconds, then run and walk alternately.

There is a cardiovascular training level for each individual below which the system is not stimulated sufficiently to produce a training effect. If you fall below that level, as you would if you sat down to rest, you've wasted a lot of effort; the time you're below isn't doing you any good, because you're not getting a training stimulus. Nor are you gaining anything from the energy you spend to get back up to the level that does you good. So the trick is to orchestrate your activity in such a way that the slow periods give you enough of a rest to be able to maintain vigorous activity in the fast periods, without being so inactive that you're penalizing yourself.

In interval training, you can work longer without fatigue because these brief periods of active rest allow for the reconversion of lactic acid and other metabolites, so that they don't limit your performance. You'll be doing more physical work and putting more of a load on your circulo-respiratory system after interval training than you will after continuous distance training. You can stand a heavier load in interval training because you haven't let your metabolic waste products pollute the working mechanisms of your body.

During your endurance lope in the first eight weeks, you worked to sixty percent of maximum. Now we're going to speed you up so that your Training Pulse Rate goes to seventy percent of maximum during the fast portions of the six-minute period.

Start out—running in place, jogging, Fitness Hopping, dancing—at your old loping rate for thirty seconds.

In the next thirty seconds, speed up your motion to an extent that raises your pulse rate to seventy percent of maximum training rate. It will take a few tries to find out what effort is required to achieve that result. You know basically that if you go faster, your heart rate will increase. How much faster is something your body will teach you by the second or third session.

Now a minute has passed. In the next thirty seconds, slow your activity, giving yourself a rest, but not to such an extent that your heart rate falls below your loping pulse rate. In other words, if you were doing your loping workout at a pulse rate of 110, let your pulse lower to that rate during this active rest interval.

After thirty seconds of active rest, speed up for thirty seconds of intensive exercise. Then slow down. Then speed up. And so forth, for six minutes.

Reminder: Take your pulse after two minutes. Don't exceed your Training Pulse Rate—seventy percent of the difference between 220 and your age. At the same time, don't be alarmed if you haven't quite made it to your Training Pulse Rate after two minutes. It may take another interval of intensive exercise to do that. After the fourth minute, take your pulse again during your active rest interval. If you're too high, don't move so fast during your next thirty-second intensive exercise burst. If you're too low, move faster.

Even if you miss your Training Pulse Rate by ten beats per minute or so for several sessions, it's no big deal. Eventually you'll find the target. Toward the end of your second eight-week period, you'll be moving a lot faster to produce your Training Pulse Rate than you were at the beginning. When that begins to happen, you're really getting in shape.

STEP THREE

Now we're going to put more quality into your program. And we're going to perfect the element of *relaxation.*

We're moving up to eighty percent of all-out effort. These are energetic, fast workouts. "Energetic" and "fast" imply relaxation. You can't move well with your brakes on. You can't get speed unless you're relaxed. Excess tension acts as a brake on the body's ability to perform work.

Some of the muscles are prime movers. Others are antagonists to the work you're going to perform. You have to let the antagonists relax while you're using the prime movers to get the work done.

Muscle Strengthening

You've got muscle mass. You've got muscle endurance. The final ingredient is muscle strength.

We've already seen some increase in strength during the previous periods. Inevitably, the exercises you've done have made once dormant muscles stronger. But to bring muscle strength up to a respectable level, you've got to do exercises designed for that purpose. Remember, you can't work effectively for mass, endurance and strength at once. You can only work for one at a time.

Basically, training for strength takes less time than building for bulk or endurance. You achieve strength by using heavier loads and fewer repetitions. These exercises take only two minutes out of our ten-minute program, leaving eight minutes to complete our circulo-respiratory endurance training.

1. Strength Pushaways

Once again, the first exercise for muscle strength is the pushaway. But the exercise takes on decidedly different characteristics. For the endurance pushaway, we went back to the wall to make things easier, so that we could get forty pushaways. Now we want to make things so difficult that we can get no more than five. So we not only go to the floor, we have to make some adjustments.

There are two basic ways to make the exercise more difficult. The first is to elevate the feet—placing them on a chair, or a stair, or a table, or even against the wall. The second way is to have someone put his hand on your back while you do your pushaway, just firmly enough so that you can't get more than five. You can guide him to the proper pressure; he'll find it quickly enough.

Ideally, you would make the exercise so difficult that you could do only one. With the same degree of difficulty, you would then try to train up to five. Then you'd intensify it even further.

2. Strength Sitbacks

Same position as for earlier sitbacks—on the floor, feet hooked to a piece of furniture, knees drawn up.

Now assume a position you can hold without trembling for *only five seconds*. After five seconds, let yourself go down to the floor, and rest.

There are two basic ways to create that much difficulty for yourself. The first is to extend your arms over your head. The second is to hold a weight either in your hands or in your arms, folded across your chest. Obviously, a deep sitback may very well be enough at first to give you a good challenge for five seconds. But if it isn't, try your arms in different positions. If that isn't enough, add weight. A heavy dictionary or encyclopedia or a cast-iron pot from the kitchen (even the lid at first) will do.

When you've finished your strength sitback, do another set of strength pushaways. Then another sitback, another pushaway, another sitback. Three times for each exercise, alternating.

You're going to be falling all over the place at the outset. Don't worry about it. It's only for two minutes. It may seem arduous, but it's also amusing. What's remarkable is that by the third week you'll be doing harder things than those you were unable to do in the first week.

You'll feel it when you've given a sufficient effort: it's at the onset of trembling of your abdominal muscles. No need to go beyond that. The effort of the first week will be insufficient for the third week to give you a strength workout, because you're getting stronger. Once again, you'll feel it and make the necessary adjustments.

Reminder: Don't exceed your Training Pulse Rate. It's now eighty percent of 220 minus your age. That's high enough.

Cardio-respiratory Sprint Intervals

In the next eight minutes we'll use a more energetic form of interval training.

At eighty percent of maximum, a fifty- to sixty-year-old person by this point can exercise at a Training Pulse Rate of 130. A forty-year-old person can go to 140.

To achieve these levels, you're going to shorten your sprinting level to fifteen seconds.

Start your activity at your Training Pulse Rate during the second eight weeks. Move at that rate for fifteen seconds. Then, in the next fifteen seconds, move at whatever rate is required to work your Training Pulse Rate up to the appropriate eighty percent level.

From then on, alternate slow and fast periods each fifteen seconds for eight minutes.

Again, it will take two to three minutes to work your heart rate up to your goal. Take your pulse after two minutes, four minutes and six minutes and make the appropriate adjustments.

Reminder: Again, the key to activity at this level is relaxation. Recall your relaxation exercises when you attempted to lower your resting pulse rate. Before starting your program, try to loosen up in the same manner. Sink your weight into a chair, let your feet grow heavy on the floor, let your shoulders fall naturally to the sides, unclench your teeth, unfurrow your brow, relax your eyes. Practice belly breathing. Let a hand ride on the belly, making sure that it moves out when a breath is drawn in. The hand and the belly fall when the breath is exhaled. Pause and relax for a moment at the end of each exhalation.

While you're exercising, practice this method of dynamic relaxation: Begin with a normal amount of tension. Then deliberately increase the tension, first by imagining that little bears are grabbing hold of your ankles, then by exaggerating your muscular contractions and imagining that a big bear is grabbing you and pulling you back. When you are very tense, shake off the bear, relax your muscles and let the tension go. The objective is to get below the level of tension with which you began.

ACQUIRING TOTAL FITNESS

Step One:	Tissue rebuilding and cardiovascular reconditioning, first eight weeks
Minutes	**Exercise**
0–1	Limbering warmup: reach, twist, bend, turn (pages 212-14)
1–2	15–20 pushaways (pages 215-17)
2–3	Sitbacks held for 15–20 seconds (pages 217-22)
3–4	Repeat pushaways
4–5	Repeat sitbacks
5–10	Continuous lope at 60% pulse (pages 222-24)
	Cool-down stroll
Step Two:	Muscular endurance and cardiovascular reconditioning, second eight weeks
	Limbering warmup
0–1	40–50 pushaways (fast)
1–2	Sitbacks held for 40–50 seconds each

2–3	Repeat pushaways
3–4	Repeat sitbacks
4–10	Endurance intervals (30-second lope intervals alternated with 30 seconds of active rest at 70% pulse)
	Cool-down stroll

Step Three:	Muscular strength and cardiovascular reconditioning, third eight weeks
	Limbering warmup
0–2	Alternate 1–5 pushaways with sitbacks held 1–5 seconds
2–10	Sprint intervals (15-second lope intervals alternated with 15 seconds of active rest at 80% pulse)
	Cool-down stroll

MAINTENANCE

You're fit now. You can start thinking about what you're going to do with all the qualities you've gained. Up until this point, the exercise has been done solely for the purpose of getting the foundations built. Now that they're built—and they are —you can direct the effort in specific ways; for example, how to increase abilities in whatever sports or other recreational activities give you pleasure. You're ready to move full bore into your specialty. You're ready to play.

You'll be astonished at how much more pleasure you get out of sport. If you play three times a week, that's probably enough to keep you in shape—assuming that you adhere faithfully to your five daily minimum-maintenance requirements:

stretching, two hours of standing, overload lifting, a three-minute elevated pulse rate, and a 300-calorie burn-off.

But if you can't play—or if you want to be certain that you'll maintain the level of fitness you've reached—you should keep up your ten-minute, three-days-a-week workouts. These will maintain a satisfactory level of muscle tissue development, muscular endurance and strength, and cardio-respiratory endurance. Here are three such maintenance workouts:

A

Minutes	Exercise
0–1	Limbering warmup
1–1.5	5 strength pushaways
1.5–2	Strength sitback, held 5 seconds each
2–10	Endurance lope (continuous at 80% pulse)

B

Minutes	Exercise
0–1	Limbering warmup
1–2	20 expansion pushaways
2–3	Expansion sitbacks held 20 seconds each
3–10	Endurance intervals (30 seconds of rapid circulo-respiratory exercise alternated with 30 seconds of "active rest," such as walking or slow pedaling, for 7 minutes at 80% pulse)

C

Minutes	Exercise
0–1	Limbering warmup
1–3	50 endurance pushaways
3–5	Endurance sitbacks held 50 seconds each
5–10	Sprint intervals (15 seconds of rapid circulo-respiratory exercise alternated with 15 seconds of "active rest," for 5 minutes at 80% pulse)

XII

Finishing Touches

Now that you're fit for a more active life, you have the capacity to accomplish some objectives that were formerly beyond your reach. You can perfect your body further by correcting any specific problems that might be giving you physical or psychological discomfort. And you can get in top condition for recreational sports such as bowling, swimming, golf, softball, tennis or skiing.

Each objective requires a special exercise beyond those you've been doing.

Because problems would interfere with the playing of sports, we'll consider them first.

SPECIAL PROBLEMS

A program of general fitness will help every part of your body, but some parts may need extra attention. The rule applies: Use makes the organ. It becomes what you make of it.

There are three special problem areas: the back, the waistline, and hips and thighs.

The back. Most of us have felt the twinge of pain in the lower back that signals problems ahead. It may be due to the natural erosion of tissue, or to misuse or disuse.

Standing for any length of time can cause discomfort for the person with low-back problems. That's usually because he puts himself in a poor position. The general rule is never to stand or move in a manner that requires an increase in the curvature of the lower back. That means no arching of the back, no leaning backward, no backbends. Often a person standing for a long time in one place will, at some point, put his hands behind him. That exaggerates his lordotic curve and puts the weight of his upper body exactly where he doesn't want it. The lordotic curve is located precisely where the back of a secretarial chair hits you. This chair is supposed to assist posture. In fact it's antiposture; it's accentuating the problem.

The best seated position is not a rigid one. It's a comfortable slouch. A pillow on your chair at the base of your spine is extremely helpful. If you can put your feet on an ottoman, you're ahead of the game. In any case, try to keep one foot higher than the other at all times. And keep changing positions. Never stay in the same position for very long.

There are two simple exercises to do each day. In the first, lie on the floor, bring your knees to your chest and, with the aid of your hands, draw the knees in just so far that you can feel your lower spine on the floor. Hold that position for five seconds.

The second exercise is the pelvis raiser. Lie on your back with your hands under your buttocks. Draw your feet up with the soles together. Tilt the pelvis upward off the floor, press the small of the back down against the floor and hold for five seconds. Work up to ten seconds.

Backstroke swimming is excellent therapy for back problems. And if you have access to a gym, pulldowns on a "lat" machine, a pulley device with weights, are enormously helpful. Sit on a bench under the bar, grasp the bar with both hands, and pull just enough to raise the weight slightly off its platform. Then bend from side to side five to ten times. Next, rotate the bar as far as it will go in both directions. Do this five to ten times. Finally, pull the bar down alternately behind and in front of your head five to ten times. Caution: Never do these exercises while kneeling. Always sit on a bench. Also, avoid exercises that compress the spine, such as lifts, presses or standing curls.

When you walk, it's important to straighten your lower back in order to reduce the excess curve in your spine. You can do this by concentrating on your navel or your belt buckle. Try to walk with it as high off the ground as possible. At the same time, lift the chest up just a fraction of an inch. That puts the shoulders where they belong. In that posture, each step becomes a corrective exercise.

Flabby waistline. Are you sure it's flabby? Frequently, members of the club where I play golf come up to me in the locker room and ask how they can get rid of their potbellies. "That'll take about two seconds," I tell most of them. "What else do you want?"

The potbelly, universally considered to be the first sign of deterioration, is usually a consequence of bad posture. For proof, go to a mirror and observe yourself from the side. The chances are about ninety-eight percent that you'll see a pot. What's happened is that the bowl formed by your pelvic bones has spilled forward, and the viscera—commonly called the gut—are pressing against the stomach wall. Now if you raise both your navel and your breastbone slightly, the anterior portion of the pelvis will be lifted, the bowl will become level again, and the viscera will settle back into it. Presto, a good portion of your potbelly will be gone.

I'll never forget my friend the professor of Spanish whose wife came to me with a tale of woe about the erosion of their sex life. He was a mess, all right. He had no meat on his shoulders, a poor posture and a potbelly. Because of his pot, he was trying to lose weight. Due to his diet restriction he was obviously malnourished. The reason he was willing to agree to see me was his appearance. As he told me, "When I look in the mirror, I remember how I looked ten years ago, and I'm ashamed." What shamed him most was all the "fat" he was accumulating around his midsection.

We got rid of his potbelly in two seconds. He was so elated that he turned to his fitness program with a vengeance.

Naturally, we can set you up in the right posture, but we can't keep you there. To do that requires an effort on your part. The best exercise you can do is the sitback you learned in your fitness program. In addition, you can consciously endeavor to improve the tone of your abdominal wall by making an exercise of standing or walking. There's only one healthy standing posture; the corrections you employ to cure your back problems are the same ones you use to combat your pot. Elevate the chest a fraction, and let your shoulders fall naturally to the sides. Your head will come naturally to a balanced position on your shoulders. Now lift your navel—or your belt buckle—as high off the ground as you comfortably can.

The abdomen is a holding muscle. It should be exercised in the position for which it's designed. Every time you walk, take ten steps with your abdomen hard. As you do, probe your abdominal musculature with your fingers to make the belly stay hard. Tense, then relax. You'll find it quite an effort at first. But gradually you'll be able to increase the number of steps. Don Ameche, the actor, walks an hour and a half with a tight belly every day of his life.

In the French Army, they put a coin between the buttocks of a recruit and make him march around without dropping the money. You don't have to go to such extremes. A better way is to imagine that you have a beautiful bushy tail. You wouldn't want it to knock things over, or get dirty. So you tuck it between your legs.

Good posture can't be achieved by five minutes

of exercise. It's a consequence of how you hold yourself during the day. Use makes the organ. The longer you keep trying to change, the more likely that change will occur. Four hours of gentle attention are infinitely more valuable than five minutes of violent exercise.

Flabby hips and thighs. A common problem for women. In addition to your fitness program, you can do the following exercise. Lie on one side, then raise and lower the top leg as fast as possible, until you can no longer maintain the speed— twenty to sixty times. Rest and repeat. Alternate sides. Rest and repeat.

A second good exercise is to lunge forward with extra long strides. This exercise can be done in place. Do one leg at a time. Return to the starting position. Repeat rapidly, twenty to sixty times, or until you can't maintain the fast speed. Then alternate sides.

PERFORMANCE

When I was in high school, I tried out for all the teams. But I soon realized that I just didn't have what it took to be a fine athlete. I was tall enough. My strength and endurance seemed okay. I was limber. But I didn't have the speed, power or agility to reach varsity levels. My fitness made my failure all the more frustrating. I determined to find out what it was that I didn't have. I've been researching that question ever since.

People performing to their maximum who are seeking ways to improve their maximum are the materials for my research. My subjects have included astronauts, executives, and world-class athletes. The setting in which I now work could hardly be more ideal. *Life* once called UCLA "the Athens of sports." The university is hardly a jock school; its faculty is rated among the top ten in the country. Yet, for the last ten years, UCLA has won an almost preposterously disproportionate share of the national championships for which members of the National Collegiate Athletic Association compete. There are eighteen such championships. There are several hundred NCAA members competing for these each year. For three straight years, UCLA won four of the eighteen championships. In the past ten years, the school has won twenty-one championships.

UCLA's head trainer is one of my students. So are numbers of the world-class athletes who compete for the school. Our Human Performance Laboratory is not in the business of turning out champions, but it does have champions to study.

What we try to discover are the limiting aspects of their performance. Why can't this runner go faster? Why can't that jumper go higher? Sometimes the answers are simple. A baseball player needs to get to first base more quickly from home plate. If he can't he'll be benched. We watch his style and discover he's too uptight. We teach him to drop almost to his knees after he hits the ball and starts for first base. This lowers his center of gravity and enables him to run faster.

While the answers are most often physiological, they can be psychological as well. Years ago, when I was teaching at the University of Southern California, Jack Davis, a hurdler, came to me for help. Like all runners, he wanted to improve his time. We worked on strength and endurance, but neither was enough. Then we started working on rhythm. We taught him to think rhythm even when he wasn't running. He broke the world's record.

Sometimes we just can't solve problems. Once a potato farmer came down from Alaska to see if we could help him train for the marathon. He could run all day around the track at nine miles an hour, but when we got him to run ten miles an hour he lasted six minutes. When we tried to train him on a treadmill, he'd exhaust even faster. We never did speed him up.

But failures are the exception. Almost anyone can improve his performance at whatever sport he plays, provided he's willing to work at it and assumes a realistic attitude.

I've long since stopped worrying about my own limitation. At sixty, I'm elated to be going like fifty. I'm content to golf or bowl or cycle or play tennis or paddle my canoe. To be able to practice these sports, I first achieved an acceptable level of fitness by following a course very similar to the one I've given you. From the point where I was fit, I could substitute the sports I enjoyed for the exercise program. I do something physical every day, except on days when I don't feel well. I have to feel pretty bad not to do anything. I live in Westwood Village, just off the UCLA campus.

Each day I walk to my office and walk home again, a round trip of two miles. If I haven't time for sports, or if the weather doesn't permit, I'll either lift weights or ride a stationary bike, depending on which I need the most. This program keeps me in just enough condition so that if I want to get into better shape for something special I don't have far to go.

But I have no illusions about my program. Because I've reached a satisfactory level of fitness doesn't mean I'm specifically conditioned to take on all comers in all sports and active games. I know that any sport for which I'm not specifically conditioned—even if it's a parent-pupil softball game, or a pickup touch-football game—could put me out of action for a week. So I try to keep my recreational exertion below "heavy." I don't indulge in any heroics. And I stay pretty much with my maintenance routine and regular sport.

SPECIFICITY

If your objective is to play a sport well, you must carry your program beyond the fitness level. For sports, you must be specific.

"Specificity" means the adaptation to imposed demands. It applies to work or play. I once knew a woman in fairly decent shape who returned from a two-week skiing trip to discover that her cleaning woman had moved away. She cleaned the house herself—and strained her muscles in the process.

Her skiing fitness was no help; it wasn't specific for housecleaning.

The body responds to the way demands are placed on it. Form follows function. If you function a certain way, your body begins to take that shape. We teach swimmers to adapt to their needs by stretching their ankles so that they will bend back beyond a straight line. They do this by sitting on the ankles every chance they get. These extra-flexible ankles give them more thrust in the water.

It's important to remember that performance and fitness are separate phenomena. Two men train for the same strength event. One works twice as hard as the other on cardiovascular conditioning. His condition is twice as good. But the second man does specific conditioning for the event itself, and gives it the same amount of time the other man gives to cardiovascular conditioning. The second man is twice as fit for the event.

Anyone who has ever swum as hard and as fast and as long as he could knows that it takes strength as well as endurance and suppleness. But in studies of swimmers who do nothing but swim, we've found that their strength increases only up to a point. As the competitive season continues, it actually falls off. A varsity swimmer working four hours a day may be increasing the effectiveness of his performance, but he is losing strength in the process. In order to maintain his strength, he must do fitness exercises as well. Years ago, when I coached swimming, I was one of the first to bring weights onto the pool deck.

Getting in shape for one sport doesn't put you in

shape for another. We proved this point in an experiment with basketball players and swimmers. At the start of the season, we tested them at running and swimming. At the end of the season, when they were supposedly in fantastic shape, we tested them again. The basketball players had increased their running time but not their swimming time. The swimmers had increased their swimming time but not their running time.

At the fitness level, swimming is a marvelous activity. People seeking an adequate degree of fitness could get all the strength and endurance and flexibility they needed using swimming alone as their exercise—as long as they constantly intensified the swimming. But competitive swimmers would probably hinder their performance if they trained to be fit and fast at the same time.

If you're training for jumping, as in volleyball or basketball, you need a large amount of muscular strength, but if you develop beyond this needed amount it will not improve your jumping ability. Any further training is a waste of time and energy that would be better spent on improving the skills and strategy of the game.

Professional football players work up to a high level of fitness before the season. During the season, they do touch-up exercises such as running and weight lifting, but only enough to maintain the desired level of fitness. At the end of the season they have less strength and endurance than they had at the beginning of the season, but they have far more skill.

About the only sports in which athletes benefit

by achieving and maintaining maximum fitness are those that are pure fitness in character, such as shot-putting and running. For most others, fitness won't help beyond a certain point.

The person whose hobby is fitness, who devotes four to six hours a day to lifting weights, isn't harming his health. But beyond a certain level he's making neither health nor performance gains.

SPECIFIC TRAINING FOR SPORTS

Training for a particular sport is a program in itself, above and beyond programs to achieve minimum-maintenance levels or reserves of fitness. It requires a complete analysis of the activity. It takes place in a systematic process. If excellence is the objective, it's a year-round program.

The best single way to train for a sport is to practice the sport itself. But even twice-daily practice of the sport won't bring you anywhere near the peak of your capacity.

To achieve fitness for an event is a process so arduous that it's best left to young athletes. It involves training for long and brief endurance, coordination and flexibility, acclimatization, heat tolerance, orthostatic tolerance, anti-gravity adjustments, tension reduction and strength contraction. But while developing the systems of the body for competition is esoteric and complex, training for each aspect of the sport itself is something any player can do.

The dimension of the sport must first be defined. From this definition comes the structure of the program. The dimensions are time, distance, force, posture, skill and concentration.

Since tennis is currently America's fastest-growing sport, we'll use it as a model.

Time. We must establish the duration and frequency. How long is the match? How many matches will you play in a day or a week?

Three sets of tennis are an ordinary match. Each set takes about thirty minutes. The sets are theoretically continuous, but in social tennis the players frequently give way to others after each set. We'll assume, however, that the play is continuous, because you have to be conditioned for that eventuality.

Play varies between very active and moderately active. A match may last two hours, but there will be periods of relative calm before and after intensive stress during a prolonged rally or point.

How do you train for this? Continuous jogging for an hour and a half or making a series of mile or half-mile runs would not be specific for tennis. The right training would correspond to the event: episodes of running interspersed with periods of rest.

If each set is thirty minutes, the proper program would be to train for thirty minutes, sit for a few minutes, then resume. During the running periods, there should be intervals of up to one minute of fast running, broken by periods of slow jogging. The spurts should be as fast as you can go. You wouldn't have to worry about exhausting yourself;

the knowledge that you're going to have to keep this up for half an hour would limit your effort. During the half hour, your pulse should never go below 120 beats, or seventy percent of your maximum performance.

That's the general idea, but you should tailor the exercise to your knowledge of your own game. If you're a steady hitter who gets into prolonged rallies of a minute, then you train for a minute. If your rallies are almost never more than thirty seconds, then train for thirty seconds. The best way to determine your needs is to observe your own game the next time you play. If during the course of half an hour of tennis you have seven extremely long points lasting a minute, then during your half hour of training you should spurt at least seven minutes.

Distance. Once again, we operate on the principle that the workout should resemble the match itself if you want to train for your maximum.

During the thirty-minute training program, do short, rapid distance moves in different directions. Hop half a dozen times, then move quickly to the right four or five steps, hop again, then move to the left. Move backward and forward, and side to side. Move in a box if you wish. These movements approximate the distances you run to retrieve your opponent's shot.

Force. The best specific exercise is to strengthen your grip. You can do this by squeezing an old tennis ball. But a better method is to get a hand spring that you can just barely close, and try to close it four or five times. You can exert more force on the object in your nonplaying hand at the same time.

Early in the season, you want to build up the tissues in the elbow to avoid injury. Tennis elbow is of mysterious origin, but we know that it has to do with tendons, muscles and their nerve supply. One preventive procedure is to build up the thickness and strength of the muscles in the elbow and the ligaments in the elbow region so that they're less apt to tear under strain. We do this with fifteen to twenty executions of elbow flexion, such as curls with a barbell or dumbbell. Pushups are very good. So are chinups. In these exercises, "load to fifteen and build to twenty." In other words, use as much weight as will give you a moderate workout at fifteen executions. Then try to work up to twenty. Once there, increase the weight, or the difficulty of the position.

All of these exercises include the shoulder joint as well as the elbow joint, which is excellent, because there's a theory that the locus of the elbow injury might be in the shoulder region.

For endurance, swing your racket, simulating forehand, backhand, smash and serve. Squat for ground strokes, reach for smashes. One set of twenty to sixty strokes. If you have access to a gym, simulate the strokes on a pulley machine.

Skill. Break the movements into their smallest components. Example: Practice taking the racket back before you practice the forward stroke. Put the parts back together as soon as you can. While practicing each part, try to keep the tempo at game speed.

Posture. All of the special exercises we're using to develop muscle and ligament bulk, and muscular endurance are performed in the posture of tennis.

Tennis is an upright sport, but it should be played in a crouched position, with only occasional moments of full stretch and reach. This tells us that the training exercises should all be performed either in the crouch or in a wholly upward, extended position.

Concentration. It's a product of motivation and attitude. The main point is to know your environment—the court, your opponent, the referee, the crowd—and yourself. The last is the most important. The key is to remain in control of your surroundings.

THE GUIDING PRINCIPLE

Whatever the sport, exercises to better performance should be performed in the same posture with the same intensity and rhythm inherent in the event. The athlete should determine the important phases of the motion, the ranges of motion and the joint angles of the limbs during the event.

Here are some special conditioning exercises for the most popular sports:

Bowling. Arm swinging, using a bowling ball. One set of twenty to sixty executions.

Forward lunging, simulating delivery. One set of twenty to sixty.

Swimming. Ankle stretching. Sit on the ankles.

Bend and rotate the trunk while sitting on the ankles. Four sets of ten to twenty.

Lie on a cushion with your arms and legs extended. Hold two cans of soup and do swimming motions with the arms and legs. Two sets of twenty to sixty.

Tennis. Practice your strokes with your tennis racket. Reach for serves and smashes. Dart into position for difficult forehands and backhands. Punch out a few net shots. Keep this going at game speed for a couple of minutes.

Squeeze two tennis balls, one in each hand, as hard as you can for a slow count of ten. Relax. Repeat three times.

Golf. Simulate the golf swing while holding a can of soup in your left hand. One set of twenty to sixty.

Put a club against your back, in a horizontal position. Hold it there with your arms, and twist your trunk. Two sets of twenty to sixty.

Softball. Swing a bat. One set of twenty to sixty.

Circle your arm while holding a ball. One set of twenty to sixty.

Skiing. Side-jump over a low barrier, with your feet together as though they were tied. One set of twenty to sixty.

Standing, put your back against the wall as if you were sitting in a chair. Hold the position for thirty seconds. Increase gradually to sixty seconds. Then try it on one leg.

Whether your objective is to correct specific physical problems or improve your performance in sport, you can do so by adding a few special exercises to your three-times-per-week maintenance program. Do them either with your regular workouts or on alternate days, whichever is more convenient.

It's best to take *one* objective at a time. Work on it until you're in shape, then take on another one. Trying to cure a weak back, develop a trimmer waist and thighs, and acquire fitness for sports all at once is asking for trouble. Take it easy, and you'll have it all.

ABOUT THE AUTHORS

Laurence E. Morehouse, Ph.D., is professor of exercise physiology and founder and director of the Human Performance Laboratory at the University of California at Los Angeles. He is the author of the sections on exercise and physical conditioning in the *Encyclopaedia Britannica,* the *Encyclopedia Americana,* the *Encyclopedia of Sports Medicine* and the *Encyclopedia of Physical Education.* His book *Physiology of Exercise* is in its seventh edition, and is the standard text for colleges and universities throughout the world. In 1968, the National Academy of Science selected him to deal with metabolic problems of astronauts in their exploration of the moon's surface.

Leonard Gross wrote for *Look* for twelve years as a senior editor, Latin American correspondent, European Editor and finally West Coast Editor. He has published more than 300 magazine articles and six books. He is currently at work on a novel, a film and a series for television.